McGRAW-H...

M000220090

Pocket Guide to Lung Function Tests

2nd Edition

Bob Hancox

BSc, MD, MRCP (UK), FRACP

Respiratory Physician

Waikato Hospital, Hamilton, and University of Otago,
Dunedin, New Zealand

Ken Whyte

MD, FRCP (Glasgow), FRACP

Consultant Respiratory Physician

Auckland City Hospital and Greenlane Hospital,
Auckland, New Zealand

The McGraw·Hill Companies

Sydney New York San Francisco Auckland
Bangkok Bogotá Caracas Hong Kong
Kuala Lumpur Lisbon London Madrid
Mexico City Milan New Delhi San Juan
Seoul Singapore Taipei Toronto

First published 2001
Reprinted 2003

Second edition
Text © 2006 Bob Hancox and Ken Whyte
Illustrations and design © 2006 McGraw-Hill Australia Pty Ltd
Additional owners of copyright are acknowledged on the Acknowledgments page.

National Library of Australia Cataloguing-in-Publication data:

Hancox, Bob.
McGraw-Hill's Pocket guide to lung function tests

2nd ed.
Bibliography
Includes index.
ISBN 0 074 71596 8.

1. Pulmonary function tests. I. Whyte, Ken. II. Title.
III. Title: Pocket guide to lung function tests.

616.24075

Published in Australia by
McGraw-Hill Australia Pty Ltd
Level 2, 82 Waterloo Road, North Ryde NSW 2113
Acquisitions Editors: Meiling Voon and Thu Nguyen
Production Editor: Kathryn Murphy
Editor: Caroline Hunter
Proofreader: Tim Learner
Indexer: Glenda Browne
Designer (cover and interior): Lara Scott, Unhinged Productions
Illustrator: Alan Laver, Shelly Communications
Typeset in Sabon 8.5/11 by Anne McLean, Jobs on Mac
Printed on 80 gsm woodfree by CTPS, Hong Kong.

The McGraw·Hill Companies

Contents

Preface

*'Air goes in and out, blood goes round and round, oxygen
is good.'*
(physiology for surgeons, author unknown)

You don't have to be a physiologist to understand that lung function
is important. If you can't breathe, none of the other organ systems will
work very well. Many patients have breathing difficulties. In these
patients, lung function tests can be used to measure how much air
'goes in and out' of these patients and how much oxygen is getting
through. They can help to establish the diagnosis and assess the severity of the condition. Unfortunately, books on respiratory physiology
tend to be stuffed with equations on gas laws and pulmonary mechanics which only the specialist can hope to remember. Few offer a
simple approach to the understanding and interpretation of *clinical*
tests of respiratory function.

   The stimulus to write this book was our impression that many students, doctors and nurses find the existing books intimidating.
Having been put off the subject by a plethora of equations, they often
fail to grasp the fairly simple concepts that underpin most lung function tests. This book is based upon the premise that the commonly
used tests of lung function are easy to understand and interpret. You
need to understand some simple principles and recognise basic patterns, but we don't believe you need to remember all the *equations*
(maybe only the one for the A-a gradient on page 81). We don't

regard this as a 'dumbing-down' of the subject—more a recognition of reality. Few clinicians have the time to develop a detailed understanding of the underlying physiological principles and even fewer use them to interpret a lung function test. If we succeed in demystifying the subject of lung function tests, we hope that you will be encouraged to read further, and we make several suggestions in the bibliography at the back of the book.

How to use this book

We have arranged this book in what we think is a logical sequence, starting with simple lung function tests and introducing more complicated tests to build on earlier concepts. We have used very few equations and little basic physiology. Some background information is provided in boxes, including a few of the dreaded equations, but these are not essential to interpreting the tests described. The intention is to cover most of the tests used in a modern lung function laboratory. At the end of each chapter there are clinical examples. Think about these before you read our interpretation of them. Our interpretation may not be best one! Results which are outside the 'normal' range are generally indicated by parentheses. We have tried to use the most common units, but there is no universal agreement on these, and those used in your local laboratory may be different.

Acknowledgments

We wish to thank our colleagues at Green Lane Hospital for their encouragement. Most of the clinical examples were provided by the pulmonary function laboratories in Green Lane Hospital and Dunedin Hospital, New Zealand, and we thank the staff of these laboratories for their help. We are particularly grateful to Dr Sze-Lin Peng and Janneke Donders for their helpful comments on the manuscript.

Some symbols commonly used in lung function tests

Gases

V = gas volume
$\dot{V}$ = gas flow
P = gas pressure
F = fractional concentration (in dry gas)
f = respiratory frequency
R = respiratory exchange ratio

D = dead space gas
I = inspired gas
E = expired gas
A = alveolar gas
T = tidal gas
B = barometric

Blood

Q = volume of blood
$\dot{Q}$ = blood flow
C = concentration or content of gas
  in blood (also compliance,
  e.g. C_L = lung compliance)
S = saturation, the percentage of Hb saturated with O_2

a = arterial blood
v = venous blood
$\bar{v}$ = mixed venous
c = capillary blood

Dash (‾) above any symbol indicates a mean value.
Dot (·) over any symbol indicates a time derivative, such as flow (volume/time).

Glossary

A-a gradient The Alveolar-arterial difference in oxygen tension. Can be easily estimated from arterial blood gases. Useful for determining whether hypoxaemia is due to hypoventilation or another process.

ATPS Ambient Temperature and Pressure Saturated with water vapour.

BTPS Body Temperature and Pressure Saturated with water vapour. The conditions inside most pulmonary function equipment resemble ATPS and measurements should be corrected to BTPS before they are reported.

CaO_2 Arterial Oxygen Content.

C_L Lung Compliance. Can be measured either as **stat**ic lung compliance (**$C_L$stat**) or **dyn**amic lung compliance (**$C_L$dyn**).

COHb CarboxyHaemoglobin.

DL_{CO} Diffusing capacity of the Lung for carbon monoxide (**CO**). Sometimes known as the transfer factor (TL_{CO}). See also K_{CO}.

eNO Exhaled Nitric Oxide.

ERV Expiratory Reserve Volume. The volume of air that can forcibly be expelled at the end of a tidal expiration. The difference between *functional residual capacity* (FRC) and *residual volume* (RV).

$FEF_{25-75\%}$ Forced Expiratory Flow between 25% and 75% of the forced vital capacity.

$FEF_{50\%}$ Forced Expiratory Flow at 50% of the forced vital capacity. See also MEF.

FER Forced Expiratory Ratio. The FEV_1/FVC ratio.

FEV_1 Forced Expiratory Volume in 1 second. The volume of air expelled during the first second of a forced maximal expiratory manoeuvre.

$FIF_{50\%}$ Forced Inspiratory Flow at **50%** of the vital capacity during a maximal inspiratory manoeuvre.

FiO_2 Fractional concentration of inspired oxygen.

FRC   Functional Residual Capacity. The volume of air in the lungs at the end of a quiet expiration, when no inspiratory or expiratory effort is being made. Sometimes known as End Expiratory Lung Volume (**EELV**).

FVC   Forced Vital Capacity. The total volume of air expelled during a forced maximal expiratory manoeuvre.

Hypoxaemia   Low oxygen content of the blood.

Hypoxia   Inadequate delivery of oxygen to the tissues.

IC   Inspiratory Capacity. The volume of air inhaled from the end of a relaxed expiration (FRC) to total lung capacity (TLC). IC, or the IC/TLC ratio, is sometimes used to estimate lung hyperinflation.

IRV   Inspiratory Reserve Volume. The extra volume of air that could be inspired at the end of a relaxed (tidal breathing) inspiration. This equals the *total lung capacity* (TLC) minus (*functional residual capacity* (FRC) plus *tidal volume* (TV)).

K_{CO} Krogh constant or DL_{CO}/VA. The ratio of the diffusing capacity to the alveolar volume. This corrects the diffusing capacity for the lung size.

MEF   Maximal Expiratory Flow. Often expressed as $MEF_{x\%}$ representing the flow where there is x% of the vital capacity remaining in the thorax. This is similar to $FEF_{x\%}$ except that for the FEF the x% refers to the percent of the vital capacity that has already been exhaled; i.e. $MEF_{75\%} = FEF_{25\%}$. Just to make things even more confusing, the term $\dot{V}max$ is often used instead of MEF such that $\dot{V}max_{25\%}$ is synonymous with $MEF_{25\%}$.

METS   Another way of expressing peak oxygen uptake during exercise testing, as multiples of the resting oxygen consumption (approximately 3.5 mL/kg/min). Not used in this book.

MIF   Maximal Inspiratory Flow. Can be expressed as $MIF_{x\%}$ representing the flow then x% of the vital capacity has already been inhaled. This is similar to $FIF_{x\%}$ except that for FIF the x% refers to the percentage of the vital capacity that remains to be inhaled; i.e. $MIF_{75\%} = FIF_{25\%}$.

MVV   Maximum Voluntary Ventilation. The theoretical maximum ventilation that can be achieved in 1 minute. Measured by asking the patient to breath 'as hard and as fast as possible' for 12–15 seconds and measuring the volume of air inspired/expired (any longer is likely to cause dizziness or syncope) and extrapolating to 1 minute. Alternatively, it can be *estimated* by multiplying the FEV_1 by 35.

Pack-years   A way of summarising a patient's smoking history. One pack-year is the equivalent of one pack of 20 cigarettes a day for 1 year. So someone who has smoked 30 cigarettes a day for 20 years has accumulated 30 pack-years of smoking.

Pa_{CO_2} The Pressure or tension of carbon dioxide in arterial blood.

PA_{CO_2} The Pressure or tension of carbon-dioxide in the Alveoli.

Pa_{O_2} The Pressure or tension of oxygen in arterial blood.

PA_{O_2} The Pressure or tension of oxygen in the Alveoli.

PC_{20} The Provocative Concentration of a stimulus (for example, methacholine) that causes a 20% fall in the FEV_1. See also PD_{20}.

P_{CO_2} The Pressure or tension of carbon dioxide. Often refers to arterial blood and is then called Pa_{CO_2}.

PD_{20} The Provocative Dose of a stimulus (such as methacholine) that causes a 20% fall in the FEV_1.

P_{O_2} The Pressure or tension of oxygen. Often refers to arterial blood and is then called Pa_{O_2}.

PEF   Peak Expiratory Flow (often, peak expiratory flow *rate*). The fastest flow obtained during a forced expiration.

Raw   Resistance to airflow in the airway. Can be standardised for the lung volume at which it was measured by multiplying Raw by the lung volume to produce the specific airway resistance (**SRaw**). See also **SGaw**.

RER   Respiratory Exchange Ratio. The ratio of carbon dioxide production ($\dot{V}_{CO_2}$) to oxygen consumption ($\dot{V}_{O_2}$). Sometimes abbreviated to **R**. Related to RQ.

RQ   Respiratory Quotient. The ratio of carbon dioxide produced to oxygen metabolised in the tissues. At steady state this equals the RER.

RV   Residual Volume. The volume remaining in the lungs at the end of maximal expiration.

Sa_{O_2} The arterial Saturation of oxygen.

SGaw   Specific airway conductance. Airway conductance (**Gaw**) is simply the reciprocal of resistance (**Raw**). Specific airway conductance is Gaw divided by the lung volume at which it was measured.

Sp_{O_2} The oxygen Saturation of arterial blood (Sa_{O_2}) estimated by Pulse Oximetry.

STPD   Standard Temperature and Pressure, Dry. $0^{\circ}C$, 760 mmHg, no water vapour.

SVC   Slow Vital Capacity. See VC.

TLC   Total Lung Capacity. The volume of air within the lungs at maximal inspiration.

TL$_{CO}$ See DL$_{CO}$.

TV   Tidal Volume. The volume of air inspired/expired in a single breath during normal breathing.

VA Alveolar Volume.

V̇A Alveolar Ventilation. Usually measured in L/min.

VC Vital Capacity. The volume of air expelled from maximal inspiration to maximal expiration during an unforced manoeuvre. In some obstructive conditions this may be greater than the forced vital capacity. Sometimes called the *slow vital capacity* (SVC) or *relaxed vital capacity*. The vital capacity can also be measured as an inspiratory manoeuvre (from maximal expiration (RV) to maximal inspiration (TLC)).

V̇CO$_2$ Carbon dioxide production. Usually measured in mL/min.

VD Volume of Dead space

VD/VT The ratio of Dead space to Tidal volume.

V̇E Minute Ventilation. The volume of air Expired in 1 minute. Equal to *tidal volume × respiratory frequency*. Measured in L/minute.

V̇max Maximal expiratory flow—see MEF.

V̇O$_2$ Oxygen uptake or consumption. Usually measured in mL/min.

V̇/Q̇ Ventilation:perfusion ratio. For alveoli or small gas-exchanging lung 'units', this refers to the ratio of ventilation (V̇) to pulmonary blood flow (Q̇). The ideal ratio is around 1. For the lungs as a whole, the concept refers to the *matching* of ventilation with perfusion such that areas of high ventilation receive a high blood flow, whereas areas of poor ventilation receive little blood flow.

VTG Volume of Thoracic Gas.

Ordering and interpreting lung function tests

Lung function tests are powerful tools in the assessment of respiratory conditions. It is probably as inappropriate to diagnose an obstructive airways disease without measuring airflow as it is to diagnose hypertension without measuring blood pressure. In addition to helping with the diagnosis, lung function tests can help to make an objective assessment of severity and monitor the response to treatment.

The lung function tests that we use in clinical practice measure just a few of the physiological variables of the respiratory system. These variables are used because they can (usually) be measured reliably, and tell us something about the function of the system in disease. The tests vary from simple spirometry, which can now be done with hand-held electronic devices, to complicated tests which require sophisticated equipment and can only be performed by a lung function laboratory. Most laboratories provide an interpretation of the results with their report. However, like most other investigations such as X-rays and blood tests, it is better if the clinician is able to add his or her own interpretation in the context of the clinical situation. It is equally important that the clinician ordering the test knows what question is to be answered. A request for 'full pulmonary function tests' will usually result in spirometry, a measurement of static lung volumes and of gas transfer, but the correct diagnosis may be missed if, say, asthma is suspected and a methacholine or histamine challenge would have been more appropriate.

'Normal' values

Most lung function tests are interpreted by comparing the results with 'predicted' or reference values—some predicted values for spirometry are included at the back of the book. More complicated tests should be reported by the lung function laboratory, along with the values predicted for that patient. A number of different prediction equations are available but, although there is broad agreement between these equations, they are not identical. Most are based on surveys of select-ed European or American populations conducted several years ago using equipment no longer used today. Lung function varies with age, sex and height and these are taken into account, but it also differs to some extent with race/ethnicity and weight which are often not accounted for. The very elderly are usually underrepresented in the populations studied and there is a particular problem in studying chil-dren and adolescents in whom the 'predicted value' depends more on their developmental than chronological age (see *The effect of growth and age on lung function*). The predicted values may not accurately represent your local population, and certainly will be inaccurate for certain individuals within any population. For example Asian patients and African-Americans tend to have lower pulmonary function val-ues than predicted by reference equations based on Europeans. For many ethnic groups the normal values are unknown. An 'ethnic factor' of subtracting 12% from the predicted value is sometimes applied to all patients who are not white/European—this is far from ideal. It is important to know if this has already been applied to the predicted values on the report.

There is also poor standardisation of the 'normal' range given on reports. Sometimes two standard deviations either side of the mean predicted value is provided. Sometimes only the predicted value is given. A rule-of-thumb which works in most cases is to allow 20% either side of the predicted value (this does not apply to the FEV_1/FVC ratio or $FEF_{25-75\%}$).

In short, be cautious when interpreting tests solely in relation to the predicted values if the tests do not fall into a disease 'pattern'. Be particularly careful if the patient is from a different ethnic group to those used in the normal value surveys.

THE EFFECT OF GROWTH AND AGE ON LUNG FUNCTION

As children grow in height, their lungs grow in size. The relationship between height and lung function changes during adolescence when the rate of lung growth appears to lag behind the rate of increase in height during the growth spurt. Lung growth appears to stop around the age of 16 in girls and 18 in boys but pulmonary function may not peak until the early 20s, and can be as late as the early 30s, especially in males. Thus a single prediction equation cannot accurately describe the complex relationship between growth, development and lung function. Detecting abnormal lung function in children can be difficult and may require serial measurements taken over several months.

There is a plateau in lung function between the ages of 20 and 30. Thereafter lung function begins to decline slowly and steadily from middle age into old age. It is unclear if the deterioration accelerates in old age—it is thought that a loss of elastic tissue may lead to mild subclinical emphysema even in healthy non-smokers.

- FEV_1 declines by 30–35 mL per year.
- Vital capacity decreases while residual volume increases, leaving total lung capacity unchanged.
- Functional residual capacity also increases with age. This may leave the diaphragm at a mechanical disadvantage, particularly if there is associated loss in height of the thorax due to osteoporosis and collapse of the thoracic vertebrae.
- The diffusing capacity declines linearly with age.

Accuracy, quality control and infection control

Most of the tests described in this book will be performed in a pulmonary function laboratory by adequately trained staff using well-maintained and calibrated equipment with proper attention to infection control. Spirometry and flow-volume loops can be performed outside the laboratory at the bedside, in clinics and elsewhere by many different health professionals. The same meticulous attention to technique, maintenance/calibration of equipment and infection control is required.

The chance of spreading infection during lung function testing is low and almost any patient can undergo tests without putting staff or other patients at risk. However, it is essential that the laboratory is

informed about infectious patients so that appropriate procedures can
be followed. These vary from laboratory to laboratory and with the
infectivity of the individual patient. For example, patients with open
tuberculosis may be scheduled for the end of the day so that the
equipment can be sterilised immediately afterward.

Chapter 1
Spirometry

Spirometry is a measure of airflow and lung volumes during a forced expiratory manoeuvre from full inspiration. It is the simplest of all respiratory function tests. It is fundamental to the diagnosis and assessment of airways disease and is often the only necessary test. The measurements made during spirometry are sometimes referred to as 'dynamic lung volumes'.

Correct interpretation of spirometry requires that it be performed correctly (see ATS/ERS criteria for acceptable and repeatable Spirometry). To obtain an accurate recording the subject should be told to:

- sit up straight
- get a good seal around the mouthpiece of the spirometer
- rapidly inhale maximally ('breathe in all the way')
- without delay, blow out as hard and as fast as possible ('blast out')
- continue to exhale ('keep going … keep going') until the patient can blow no more. In practice this is when less than 25 mL has been exhaled over 1 second. Expiration should continue for at least 6 seconds (3 seconds in children under 10 years old) and up to 15 seconds if necessary (some patients will find this exhausting and prolonged manoeuvres should be used with caution)

Manoeuvres are repeated until at least three technically acceptable manoeuvres (no coughs, air leaks, false starts) are completed. If required, more tests should be done to try to meet repeatability criteria (no more than 8 attempts in total).

The two largest FEV_1 measurements and the two largest FVC measurements should be within 150 mL of each other. The largest of each of these (not necessarily from the same manoeuvre) should be reported.

Efforts interrupted by coughing should be discarded (some patients cough only towards the end of the manoeuvre—this may not significantly alter the FEV_1 or FVC).

Poor measurement technique can produce results which mimic disease patterns. Common errors occur when the patient fails to inhale fully before the test, stops blowing too early (apparent restrictive defect), or doesn't blow out hard enough (apparent obstructive defect). Some patients are unable to perform repeatable spirometry—this may be useful information in itself. It is recommended that no more than eight blows are attempted at any one time. If reproducible results are not obtained, the highest of the technically acceptable results should be reported with a comment that repeatability criteria were not met.

Most modern spirometers can produce flow-volume loops. Inspection of the flow-volume loop, if available, will help to decide whether the measurement was done correctly as well as confirming the presence of an abnormality (see Chapter 2).

Abnormal spirometry may be masked by treatment. Bronchodilator and other relevant drugs should be withheld for at least the expected duration of action of the drug. If this is not possible, the fact should be recorded and the results interpreted accordingly.

There are several types of spirometer. Many are designed for use outside of the lung function laboratory and some are intended for home use by the patient. All types are acceptable, provided that they meet or exceed the minimum standards of the American Thoracic Society and European Respiratory Society (see *Types of spirometer*, p. 4).

FEV_1, FVC and FER

Spirometry provides three basic measurements:
- the forced vital capacity (FVC)
- the forced expiratory volume in one second (FEV_1)
- the ratio of the FEV_1/FVC (the forced expiratory ratio FER, also known as the $FEV_1\%$).

AMERICAN THORACIC SOCIETY/EUROPEAN RESPIRATORY SOCIETY CRITERIA FOR ACCEPTABLE AND REPRODUCIBLE SPIROMETRY

The ATS and ERS have recently produced joint guidelines for performing spirometry. Differences from earlier guidelines are minor. Many spirometers have built-in warnings if the acceptability criteria are not met. Some patients cannot produce acceptable and repeatable manoeuvres and you should exercise clinical judgement whether to accept an imperfect result that provides some information or discard the results of all the manoeuvres and get no information.

ACCEPTABILITY CRITERIA

- Free from artefacts (such as cough or glottis closure early in expiration)
- Free from leaks
- Good starts
  - extrapolation back from the peak flow (which is the steepest part of the spirogram curve) produces a theoretical start time from which the measurements should be timed. This 'new time zero' should occur within 5% of the FVC or within 150 mL
- Acceptable exhalation
  - Adults: at least 6 seconds of exhalation and a plateau in the volume curve (plateau = no detectable change in volume over 1 second)
  - Children aged under 10: at least 3 seconds of exhalation and a plateau in the volume curve

REPEATABILITY CRITERIA

- Three acceptable manoeuvres (meeting above criteria)
- The two largest FVC measurements within 150mL of each other
- The two largest FEV_1 measurements within 150mL of each other

When both acceptability and repeatability criteria are met, the test can be concluded. Up to 8 manoeuvres should be performed until the criteria are met or the patient is unable to continue. As a minimum, the three satisfactory (or best) manoeuvres should be saved.

All three are needed to interpret spirometry. A normal spirogram is shown in Figure 1.1 (p. 5). This plots the total volume exhaled against time. The trace becomes flat after about 3–4 seconds because the total volume of air which can be exhaled (the FVC) is expelled within this time. Approximately 80% of this volume (slightly lower

TYPES OF SPIROMETER

There are numerous spirometer devices available, and they fall into two basic categories: those measuring a change in volume, or measuring flow.

VOLUME-DISPLACEMENT SPIROMETERS

These include water-sealed devices (the original method invented by Hutchinson in the mid-1800s) in which the volume displaced is collected in a bell sealed by a water reservoir. Others may have a bellows device or rolling-seal cylinder/piston devices. The volume displaced is recorded and the flow is calculated as the volume change over time. The spirogram can be drawn by a pen (indicating volume) on moving graph paper (indicating time). More modern devices can include computer analysis of the spirogram curve. The simplicity and accuracy of these devices make them very reliable. However, each is bulky and impractical for home use.

FLOW-SENSING DEVICES

Flow-sensing spirometers measure airflow, and integrate this to determine volume. Several methods are used to detect the flow. These include pneumotachographs, in which a resistive element is placed in the airflow. The small pressure difference on either side of the element is related to the airflow. Heated wire devices use the airflow to cool a heated wire. The flow is calculated from the current required to maintain the wire temperature. Rotating vane devices place a small turbine in the airstream; the turbine spins at a rate according to the flow. Ultrasound devices measure the change in ultrasound transmission time with airflow.

Regardless of the type of device, it should be checked at regular intervals using a calibrated syringe (either 1 L or 3 L).

in older people) is exhaled within 1 second, so the FEV_1/FVC ratio is normally 0.7–0.8 or 70–80%.

Spirometry can demonstrate two basic patterns of disorder—*obstructive* and *restrictive*.

Obstructive pattern

In obstructive disorders (for example, asthma or chronic obstructive pulmonary disease), airflow is reduced because the airways narrow and the FEV_1 is reduced (Fig. 1.2). The spirogram may continue to

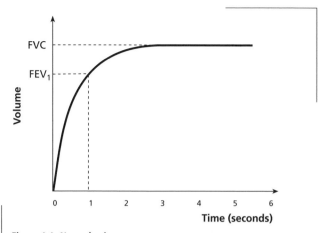

Figure 1.1 Normal spirogram
Note that approximately 80% of the total volume is exhaled in the first 1 second
(the FEV_1) and that the curve has reached a plateau by 6 seconds.

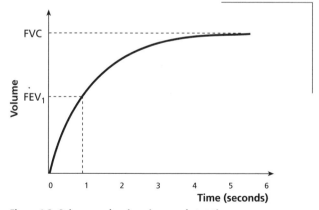

Figure 1.2 Spirogram showing airways obstruction
Both the FEV_1 and the FVC may be reduced, but the FEV_1 is reduced to a
greater extent. The FEV_1/FVC ratio is therefore low. In this patient, the forced
expiratory time is prolonged and a convincing plateau has not been reached by
6 seconds. Ideally, the patient should continue to blow until a plateau has
been reached.

rise for more than 6 seconds because the lungs take longer to empty. The FVC may also be reduced (because gas is trapped behind obstructed bronchi) but to a lesser extent than the FEV_1. Thus the cardinal feature of an obstructive defect is a reduction in the FEV_1/FVC ratio.

Although the FEV_1/FVC ratio is very useful in diagnosing airflow obstruction, the absolute value of the FEV_1 is the best measure of severity. In general, a reduction in FEV_1 to 60–80% of predicted indicates mild, 40–60% moderate and less than 40% severe obstruction.* Patients with an FEV_1 of less than 1 litre are likely to be limited by dyspnoea. If the FEV_1 is less than 0.5 litres, the patient is likely to be breathless at rest and in respiratory failure. Conversely, a patient with an FEV_1 of more than 2 litres is unlikely to be short of breath due to airways disease except on vigorous exertion.

Restrictive pattern

Restrictive disorders can be caused by disease of the lung parenchyma (such as interstitial lung fibrosis) or chest wall disease (such as kyphoscoliosis). These prevent full expansion of the lungs and therefore the vital capacity (VC or FVC) is reduced. Airflow may be normal or even increased because the stiffness of fibrotic lungs increases the expiratory pressure. Thus although the absolute value of the FEV_1 may be reduced, the FEV_1/FVC ratio is normal or high (Fig. 1.3).

A restrictive pattern on spirometry can be mimicked by a poor technique. Often the FVC is underestimated because the patient stops blowing too early. This will produce a high FEV_1/FVC ratio (Fig. 1.4). It is important to check that the spirometry was done correctly. Be cautious about diagnosing a restrictive disorder on spirometry alone, particularly if the FEV_1 is in the normal range. Clinical correlation is necessary and more detailed lung function tests are indicated. Ideally, measurement of the total lung capacity (TLC) should be used to confirm the diagnosis (see Chapter 4).

---

* There are several different ways to classify the severity of obstruction. For example, the GOLD classification of chronic obstructive pulmonary disease is based on post-bronchodilator spirometry. For patients with an FEV_1/FVC ratio <70%, mild is FEV_1 ≥80%, moderate is FEV1 = 30–80% and severe is FEV_1 <30%. (R. A. Pauwels, A. S. Buist, P. M. A. Calverley et al., 'Global strategy for the diagnosis, management and prevention of chronic obstructive pulmonary disease', *American Journal of Respiratory and Critical Care Medicine*, 2001, 163, pp. 1256–76.)

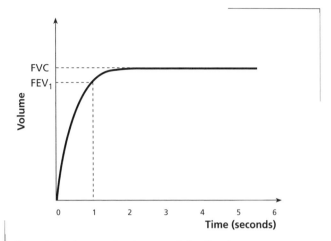

Figure 1.3 Spirogram showing a restrictive disorder
Both the FEV$_1$ and FVC may be reduced, but the FVC is reduced to the same or greater extent than the FEV$_1$. In this case the FEV$_1$/FVC ratio is high. The plateau to the curve occurs early.

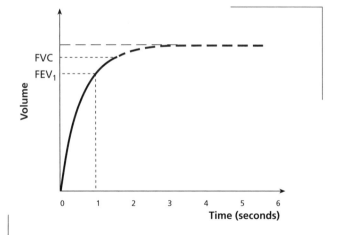

Figure 1.4 Inadequate technique mimicking a restrictive disorder
The patient stopped blowing too soon. The FVC is underestimated and the FEV$_1$/FVC ratio appears high, giving the impression of a restrictive disorder.

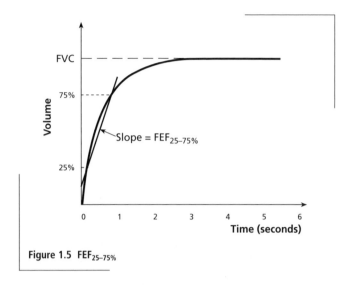

Figure 1.5 FEF$_{25-75\%}$

Other measurements of forced expiratory flow

Some spirometers will also provide other results, such as the FEF$_{25-75\%}$. This is the *forced expiratory flow* between 25% and 75% of the FVC (also called the maximum mid-expiratory flow, MMEF). This is the slope between the points on the spirogram shown in Figure 1.5. This represents the airflow in the medium and small airways. It is a sensitive but less reliable indicator of airflow obstruction than the FEV$_1$. It may indicate mild airways disease (for example, in an asthmatic who is currently stable) but has a wide range of normal values, and should be interpreted with caution if it is the sole abnormality.

Similar measurements include the FEF at fixed points of the spirogram. For example, FEF$_{25\%}$, FEF$_{50\%}$ and FEF$_{75\%}$ are the flows recorded at 25%, 50% and 75% of the FVC respectively.

In addition to the FEV$_1$, the forced expiratory volume in other time intervals may be recorded. The FEV$_{0.5}$ or the FEV$_{0.75}$ are sometimes used in children in whom the normal FEV$_1$/FVC ratio is very high. The interpretation of these measurements is similar to that of FEV$_1$ using the appropriate predicted values. FEV$_6$ (the volume exhaled in the first 6 seconds) is sometimes used as an alternative measurement to the FVC if the spirometer is unable to record beyond 6 seconds, or if the patient finds prolonged expiratory manoeuvres exhausting. The FEV_6 may underestimate the FVC in obstructive disorders, but this is unlikely to significantly alter the interpretation of the results.

Vital capacity: slow vital capacity or forced vital capacity?

In some patients with obstructive airways disease, the forced vital capacity (FVC) will underestimate the true vital capacity (VC). This is because the increase in intrathoracic pressure during the forced manoeuvre compresses airways, causing early airway closure and gas trapping. This does not happen in normal lungs. If suspected, it can be detected by measuring the vital capacity (from full inspiration to full expiration) without trying to force the air out (sometimes called a slow or relaxed vital capacity, SVC). Some pulmonary function equipment also allows the vital capacity to be measured as an inspiratory manoeuvre (inspiratory vital capacity, IVC). Slow vital capacity measurement is sometimes useful for avoiding the dizziness and syncope occasionally associated with prolonged FVC manoeuvres.

Reversibility

The reversibility of airflow obstruction is often demonstrated by repeating spirometry after treatment. Most often, a dose of inhaled beta-agonist (such as salbutamol 2.5 mg by nebuliser) is administered after the initial test and spirometry is repeated 15–30 minutes later. Other bronchodilators, such as ipratropium bromide, may also be used. Alternatively, spirometry can be repeated after a few weeks of inhaled or oral corticosteroid treatment. It is important to ensure that bronchodilators have not been taken before the initial test.

Various criteria exist for defining 'significant' reversibility. Usually an improvement of 15% or more and 200 mL or more in FEV_1 or FVC are required, since smaller changes may occur due to the variability of testing procedure and may occur by chance. In patients who are unable to perform reproducible tests, even large changes may be due to errors of measurement. Often both FEV_1 and FVC improve and the FEV_1/FVC ratio does not change. Occasionally there is a significant improvement in FVC with no change in FEV_1 and the FEV_1/FVC ratio appears to get smaller. Therefore the FEV_1/FVC ratio should not be used to assess the response to bronchodilators.

Reversibility is a characteristic feature of asthma. A significant improvement in spirometry may suggest the diagnosis of asthma even if the original measurements were within the 'normal' range. However, in chronic asthma there may be only partial reversibility of the airflow obstruction.

The airflow obstruction in chronic obstructive pulmonary disease is largely irreversible. However, a small but significant improvement in FEV_1 can be shown in many chronic obstructive pulmonary disease patients. Thus it may not be possible to distinguish between chronic obstructive pulmonary disease and chronic asthma on reversibility criteria alone. The results should be interpreted in the clinical context.

Reversibility is sometimes used to guide treatment. A large response to a bronchodilator indicates that there is a potential to improve airflow obstruction. This may justify a trial of anti-asthma medication (such as inhaled corticosteroid) in patients otherwise thought to have chronic obstructive pulmonary disease. However, a lack of response to a bronchodilator during reversibility testing does not necessarily mean that the bronchodilator will not provide important symptomatic benefits such as an improvement in exercise tolerance. The definition of significant reversibility requires that a large percentage change is needed in patients with severe airways disease. For example an improvement in FEV_1 from 0.6 litres to 0.75 litres (150 mL) would not be regarded as 'significant' because it could be due to measurement error, even though a *real* change of this magnitude may be a big improvement for the patient.

CHAPTER SUMMARY

→ Spirometry which is not performed correctly may produce misleading results.

→ The FEV_1, FVC and FEV_1/FVC ratio are all necessary to interpret spirometry.

→ An obstructive defect causes a reduction in FEV_1 and a reduced FEV_1/FVC ratio.

→ Restrictive defects cause a reduction in FVC with a normal or high FEV_1/FVC ratio.

→ 15% or more and 200 mL or more improvement in either FEV_1 or FVC after bronchodilator indicates significant reversibility. The FEV_1/FVC ratio should not be used to assess reversibility.

Clinical examples

Figures in brackets are outside the predicted range.

Patient 1A: age 31, female, European, height 1.68 m, weight 74 kg

History: Intermittent wheeze. Non-smoker.

Technician's comments: Good patient technique, results were acceptable and reproducible.

	Predicted	Measured	% predicted
FEV$_1$ litres	3.17	(2.08)	(66)
FVC litres	3.99	3.85	96
FEV$_1$/FVC %	79	54	
FEF$_{25-75\%}$ L/s	3.58	(1.14)	(32)

Spirometry was repeated 15 minutes after nebulised bronchodilator:

	Measured	% predicted	% change
FEV$_1$ litres	3.40	107	63
FVC litres	4.30	108	12
FEV$_1$/FVC %	79		
FEF$_{25-75\%}$ L/s	3.14	88	

Interpretation: There is mild airflow obstruction on initial spirometry indicated by the low FEV$_1$ and the low FEV$_1$/FVC ratio. After bronchodilator, spirometry is normal with significant improvements in the FEV$_1$ and a small improvement in FVC, indicating complete reversibility. In the context of the history, these results suggest asthma.

Patient 1B: age 50, female, European, height 1.62 m, weight 57 kg

History: Recent onset of wheeze and dyspnoea. Has smoked approximately 20 cigarettes a day for 30 years. ?Late-onset asthma.

Technician's comments: Good patient technique, results were acceptable and reproducible despite frequent cough. Patient had a cigarette 1 hour prior to being tested.

	Predicted	Measured	% predicted
FEV$_1$ litres	2.51	(1.31)	(52)
FVC litres	3.31	2.88	87
FEV$_1$/FVC %	75	45	
FEF$_{25-75\%}$ L/s	2.89	(0.52)	(18)

Spirometry was repeated 15 minutes after nebulised bronchodilator:

	Measured	% predicted	% change
FEV$_1$ litres	(1.60)	(64)	22
FVC litres	3.36	102	17
FEV$_1$/FVC %	48		
FEF$_{25-75\%}$ L/s	(0.78)	(27)	49

Interpretation: There is moderately severe airflow obstruction on initial spirometry indicated by the low FEV$_1$ and low FEV$_1$/FVC ratio. After bronchodilator, there is partial reversibility with significant improvements in both FEV$_1$ and FVC. Note that the FEV$_1$/FVC ratio does not change significantly despite the response to bronchodilator. In view of the history of smoking and the recent onset of symptoms, these results suggest chronic obstructive pulmonary disease. However, there is significant reversibility and a trial of corticosteroids to maximise lung function may be justified.

Patient 1C: age 77, male, Asian, height 1.63 m, weight 65 kg
History: Gradual onset of dyspnoea over the past year. Has smoked approximately 10 cigarettes a day for 50 years.
Technician's comments: Good patient technique, acceptable and reproducible results.

	Predicted	Measured	% predicted
FEV$_1$ litres	2.16	1.59	73
FVC litres	3.31	(1.91)	(58)
FEV$_1$/FVC %	69	83	
FEF$_{25-75\%}$ L/s	2.06	2.36	115

Interpretation: There is a restrictive pattern with a moderately reduced FVC. The FEV$_1$ is at the lower end of the normal range and the FEV$_1$/FVC ratio is high. The FEF$_{25-75\%}$ is at the upper end of the normal range, suggesting increased mid-expiratory flows despite the reduced vital capacity. Further pulmonary function tests, including lung volumes and gas transfer, would be useful in this patient—see Chapters 4 and 5. (A high-resolution CT scan later suggested pulmonary fibrosis.) Note that this patient is Asian; the predicted values given are based on Europeans, and may overestimate the 'normal' values.

Patient 1D: age 77, male, European, height 1.64 m, weight 73 kg

History: Gradual onset of dyspnoea and cough over the past few months. Has smoked approximately 20 cigarettes a day for 30 years, but gave up smoking 15 years ago. Has been treated with amiodarone for atrial fibrillation. Has a pet parrot.

Technician's comments: Good patient technique, but coughed when trying to expire fully. FVC may be underestimated.

	Predicted	Measured	% predicted
FEV$_1$ litres	2.26	2.08	92
FVC litres	3.45	2.55	74
FEV$_1$/FVC %	68	81	
FEF$_{25-5\%}$ L/s	2.10	2.09	99

Interpretation: All the measured results are within the predicted range. However, a restrictive pattern is suggested by the low/normal FVC and a high FEV$_1$/FVC ratio. The FVC may be underestimated by the patient's technique (see technician's comments). The FEV$_1$ and FEF$_{25-75\%}$ are normal and there is no evidence of airflow obstruction.

In view of the history of exposure to amiodarone and a pet bird (both of which can cause restrictive lung diseases), further pulmonary function tests, including lung volumes and gas transfer, are indicated—see Chapters 4 and 5.

Chapter 2

Flow-volume loops

S pirometry data can also be presented as a flow-volume loop. This plots airflow on the vertical axis against the total volume exhaled on the horizontal axis. Flow-volume graphs are useful because different lung disorders produce distinct, easily recognised patterns. Inspiratory manoeuvres can also be plotted on flow-volume loops and this is occasionally helpful.

The relationship between the data on the spirogram (which plots volume on the vertical axis against time on the horizontal axis) and the flow-volume loop is not immediately obvious (Fig. 2.1). Airflow on the spirogram is indicated by the slope of the curve. In effect, the flow-volume loop shows the slope of the spirogram (airflow) on the vertical axis and the volume of air exhaled on the horizontal axis. There is no direct indicator of time in a flow-volume loop and the FEV_1 cannot easily be measured from it.

By convention the flow-volume loop starts on the left of the graph at full inspiration (total lung capacity, TLC). During a forced expiration airflow rapidly rises to the *peak expiratory flow*. Flow then decreases as the volume of air remaining in the lungs decreases (Fig. 2.1). This is because the bronchi are maximally dilated at full inspiration by traction from the lung tissue. As the volume of the lungs falls, there is less traction on the bronchi and the airways narrow. In normal patients flow decreases approximately linearly with the reduction in volume and this part of the flow-volume loop is straight or slightly convex. While the peak flow is very dependent on patient effort, this latter part of the flow-volume curve is much less so. This

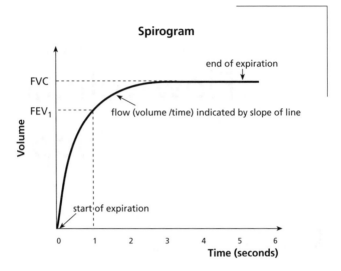

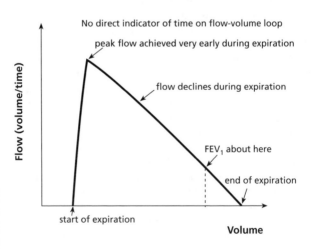

Figure 2.1 The relationship between the spirogram (volume-time graph) and the flow-volume loop

is because any extra effort increases the thoracic air pressure surrounding and compressing the airways to the same extent as the pressure driving airflow. This is known as the *effort-independent* part of the loop. It is useful to study this part of the curve because disease patterns are not mimicked by poor effort or malingering (Fig. 2.2).

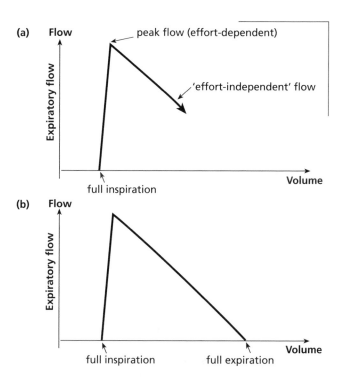

Figure 2.2 Flow-volume loops
(a) Starting from full inspiration, the flow rapidly increases to the peak expiratory flow. The flow then declines as the lung volumes fall. This section of the curve is relatively effort-independent. (b) Flow decreases linearly with lung volume until residual volume is reached (no more air can be breathed out). At the end of expiration the normal loop is approximately triangular.

(continued)

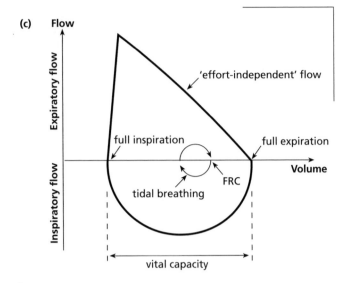

Figure 2.2 (continued)
(c) A complete inspiratory loop is approximately semicircular and should join the start of the expiratory loop at total lung capacity if there has been no air leak. The maximal flow-volume loop forms an 'envelope'. Normal breathing occurs within this envelope. The position of relaxed tidal breathing is illustrated.

The flow-volume loop can be used to assess the acceptability of spirometry manoeuvres (Fig. 2.3). Lack of an early peak suggests poor effort. Sudden tailing off of the expiratory curve suggests that the patient stopped blowing too early. Coughs are easily recognised (a loop which includes a cough may be acceptable if the overall slope is not disrupted). If the manoeuvre is completed with an inspiratory effort back to total lung capacity, a failure of the start and end of the loop to join suggests an air leak.

Obstructive pattern

In airflow obstruction the peak expiratory flow is often reduced and the maximum height of the loop is reduced. Airflow reduces rapidly

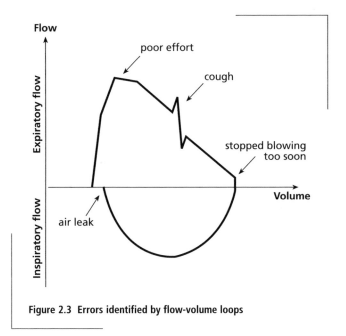

Figure 2.3 Errors identified by flow-volume loops

with the reduction in lung volumes because the airways narrow, and the loop becomes concave (Fig. 2.4(a)). This concavity of the flow-volume loop can be the first indication of airflow obstruction and may be present before the FEV_1 or FEV_1/FVC ratio become abnormal. However, it should be interpreted cautiously if it is the only abnormality. The destruction of the supporting lung tissue, as in emphysema, may allow airways to collapse during forced expiration, causing very reduced flow at low lung volumes and a characteristic 'dog-leg' appearance to the flow-volume curve (Fig. 2.4(b)).

Restrictive pattern

In restrictive disorders caused by interstitial lung disease, full lung expansion is prevented by fibrotic tissue in the lung parenchyma and the vital capacity is reduced. However, fibrotic tissue increases the elastic recoil of the lung and this may increase the airflow at a given

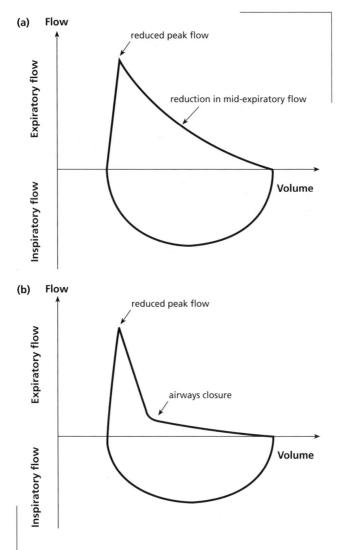

Figure 2.4 Obstructive flow-volume loops

(a) Concave loop caused by airways narrowing (for example, asthma).

(b) Airway collapse/closure, typical of emphysema.

lung volume. Thus, even though both the FEV_1 and FVC may be reduced because the lungs are small and stiff, the peak expiratory flow may be preserved or even higher than predicted. These effects make the flow-volume loop tall and narrow with a steep end-expiratory phase (Fig. 2.5).

In restrictive disorders caused by chest wall deformity or neuro-muscular disease, there is no increase in elastic recoil and, although the vital capacity is reduced, airflow, and therefore the slope of the expiratory curve, is not increased.

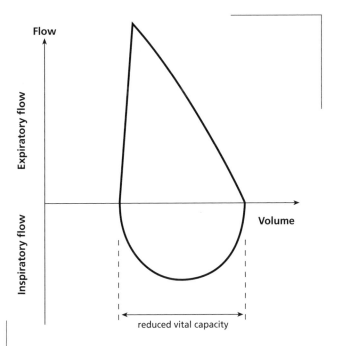

Figure 2.5 Restrictive flow-volume loop
The loop is narrow because the vital capacity is reduced, and peaked because the stiffness of the lungs increases elastic recoil and increases peak expiratory flow.

Large airway obstruction

Flow-volume loops are particularly useful in large airway obstruction (trachea or main bronchi). This reduces the peak flow rate, causing a flattening of the inspiratory/expiratory curves. There are a number of patterns, depending on the site and the variability of the obstruction (Fig. 2.6).

In *fixed obstruction* maximum airflow is limited to a similar extent in both inspiration and expiration. Both inspiratory and expiratory phases on the loop show plateaus (Fig. 2.6(a)).

In *variable extrathoracic* obstruction the obstruction worsens in inspiration because the negative pressure narrows the trachea and inspiratory flow is reduced to a greater extent than expiratory flow (Fig. 2.6(b)).

In *variable intrathoracic* obstruction the narrowing is maximal in expiration because of increased intrathoracic pressure compressing the airway, and reduced in inspiration because the intrathoracic pressure is lower than the airway pressure. Thus the flow-volume loop shows a greater reduction in the expiratory phase (Fig. 2.6(c)).

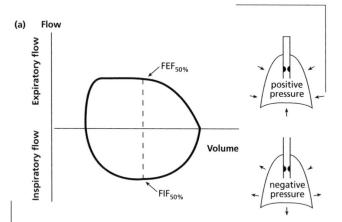

Figure 2.6 Flow-volume loops in large airway obstruction
(a) Fixed obstruction. Both expiration and inspiration are limited to a similar extent and both phases of the loop are flattened.

(continued)

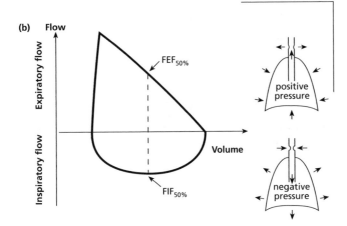

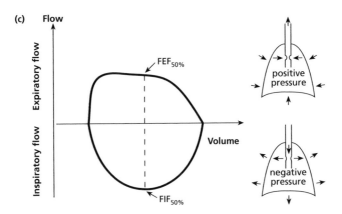

Figure 2.6 (continued)
(b) Variable extrathoracic obstruction. Inspiratory flow is reduced more than expiratory flow. The $FIF_{50\%}$ is less than the $FEF_{50\%}$. (c) Variable intrathoracic obstruction. Expiratory flow is reduced more than inspiratory flow. The $FIF_{50\%}$ is greater than the $FEF_{50\%}$.

CHAPTER SUMMARY

→ Poor effort or technique may be more obvious in flow-volume loops than in standard spirometry.

→ Small and medium airways obstruction causes a concave slope on the expiratory curve.

→ Restrictive defects due to fibrotic lung disease cause a steep slope on the expiratory curve. The loop is usually tall and thin.

→ A plateau on the expiratory or inspiratory curve or both suggests large airways obstruction.

Clinical examples

Patient 2A: age 42, female, European, height 1.65 m, weight 57.5 kg

History: Gradual onset of severe dyspnoea over 1–2 years. Ex-smoker of 30 cigarettes/day for 20 years—stopped 2 years ago.

Technician's comments: good patient technique, results acceptable and reproducible.

	Predicted	Measured	% predicted
FEV$_1$ litres	2.80	2.59	92
FVC litres	3.62	4.20	116
FEV$_1$/FVC %	77	62	
FEF$_{25-75\%}$ L/s	3.19	(1.36)	(43)

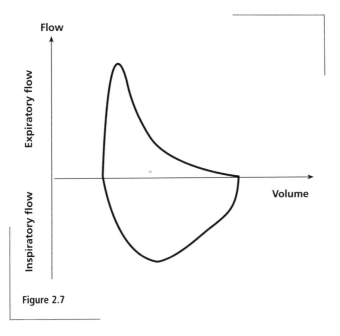

Figure 2.7

Interpretation: The FEV_1 and FVC are within the predicted range. The FEV_1/FVC ratio is low but this is mostly because the FVC is at the upper limit of normal. The $FEF_{25-75\%}$ is reduced, suggesting airflow obstruction. This is confirmed by the concave shape of the expiratory flow-volume loop. The obstructive defect appears only mild, and a further explanation for the severity of the patient's symptoms is needed.

Patient 2B: age 49, male, European, height 1.85 m, weight 68.0 kg

History: Gradual increasing dyspnoea for a few years. Smoker of 20 cigarettes a day for 30 years.

Technician's comments: good patient technique, results acceptable and reproducible.

	Predicted	Measured	% predicted
FEV_1 litres	3.89	(0.80)	(20)
FVC litres	5.34	(3.56)	(67)
FEV_1/FVC %	72	22	
$FEF_{25-75\%}$ L/s	3.74	(0.32)	(8)

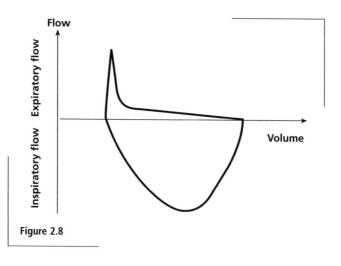

Figure 2.8

Interpretation: There is a severe obstructive defect. The FEV_1 and FVC are both low but the FEV_1 is reduced to a much greater extent and the FEV_1/FVC ratio is very low. The expiratory flow-volume loop shows a 'dog-leg' or 'L'-shape, suggesting airways collapse due to emphysema. The patient is now known to have emphysema due to smoking and alpha-1 antitrypsin deficiency.

Patient 2C: age 58, male, European, height 1.78 m, weight 95.0 kg

History: Insidious onset of dyspnoea. Ex-smoker of 15 cigarettes/day for 30 years.

Technician's comments: good patient technique, results acceptable and reproducible.

	Predicted	Measured	% predicted
FEV_1 litres	3.32	(1.75)	(53)
FVC litres	4.67	(2.54)	(54)
FEV_1/FVC %	71	69	
$FEF_{25-75\%}$ L/s	3.19	(0.97)	(30)

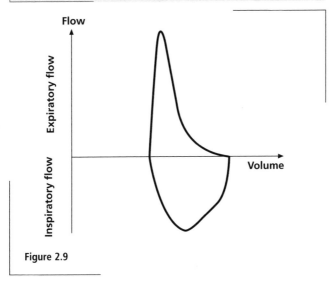

Figure 2.9

Interpretation: The FEV_1 and FVC are reduced to a similar extent. The FEV_1/FVC ratio is therefore normal. This usually indicates a restrictive abnormality. However, the mid-expiratory flow ($FEF_{25-75\%}$) is also low, possibly indicating obstruction. The expiratory flow-volume loop is tall and narrow, confirming the impression of a predominant restrictive disorder. The expiratory curve is also concave, consistent with a component of airflow obstruction. The restrictive defect needs to be confirmed by measuring lung volumes—see Chapter 4.

Patient 2D: age 38, female, European, height 1.64 m, weight 105 kg

History: Complains of 'noisy' breathing and mild shortness of breath. She has a goitre.

Technician's comments: good patient technique, results acceptable and reproducible.

	Predicted	Measured	% predicted
FEV_1 litres	2.90	2.56	88
FVC litres	3.71	3.11	84
FEV_1/FVC %	77	82	
$FEF_{25-75\%}$ L/s	3.31	2.90	88

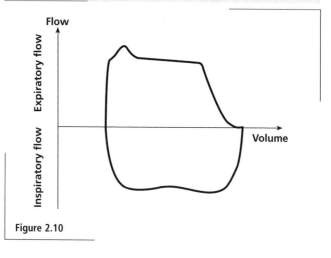

Figure 2.10

Interpretation: Spirometry is normal. The flow-volume loop is flat-tened in both the expiratory and inspiratory parts. This supports the diagnosis of fixed tracheal obstruction, presumably due to her goitre.

Chapter 3

Peak expiratory flow

Peak expiratory flow is probably the most widely used pulmonary function test. There is a variety of cheap, portable meters available for measuring peak flow at home or in the surgery. They can be invaluable for measuring day-to-day fluctuations in airway calibre in asthma. However, they have the disadvantage that the measurement of peak flow is very dependent on patient effort and technique (much more than the FEV_1 and FVC). There is also poor standardisation between different meters, and even meters of the same make may give different results. Thus, although charts of 'normal values' are widespread, these are best ignored. For monitoring asthma control it is better to compare the peak flow value to the patient's 'best' or usual measurement. For this reason all asthmatics would do well to perform occasional peak flow measurements, even when healthy, so that they have a baseline against which to assess the severity of an asthma attack. For more formal assessment of airways disease it is preferable to perform spirometry.

The peak expiratory flow is generated in the first fraction of a second of a forced expiratory manoeuvre. The major contribution to the peak flow is from the large central airways. Asthma and other obstructive diseases affecting the small airways may not be detected by measuring peak flow.

Despite its limitations peak flow measurement has a number of useful functions.

Assessment of acute asthma

Peak flow can be used to help assess the severity of an asthma attack, particularly if the measurement can be compared to the patient's best peak flow (if the best peak flow is unknown, the predicted value can be used):

- Less than 75% (children <60%) of the patient's best indicates a moderate attack.
- Less than 50% (children <40%) indicates a severe attack
- An absolute value of <100 L/min or an inability to perform a peak flow test indicate a severe attack.

Peak flow monitoring also helps to assess the response to treatment during an acute attack. A failure to improve should indicate the need for ongoing treatment and hospital admission.

Monitoring of chronic asthma

Daily (ideally twice daily) peak flow monitoring has been advocated for the routine monitoring of asthma. Large fluctuations in peak flow indicate poor asthma control. Typically there is diurnal variability, with morning peak flows being lower than afternoon or evening peak flows. Variability of more than 20% suggests persistent asthma. Variability of more than 30% indicates severe asthma.

Some patients appear to be poor perceivers of asthma symptoms. It has been suggested that regular monitoring of peak flows would provide an 'early warning' of an asthma exacerbation, allowing the patient to take preventative treatment before a severe exacerbation developed. The success of this approach is unproven. However, asthma action plans based on either symptoms or peak flows are widely used and may help patients understand and control their asthma (Table 3.1).

Diagnosis of asthma

Although spirometry is a much better test for diagnosing airflow obstruction, peak flow can be a useful aid to the diagnosis of asthma:

- If spirometry is not available, a convincing peak flow response to bronchodilator (>20% improvement) in a patient with good technique (see below) is reasonable evidence of reversible airways obstruction.

Table 3.1	Action plans should be individualised for each patient. A suggested format is shown. A number of preprepared action plan cards printed in bright colours are available

Peak flow	Symptoms	Advice
>80% of best	No change	Continue usual treatment
60–80% of best	Increasing symptoms or starting upper respiratory tract infection	Increase (or start) dose of inhaled corticosteroids
40–60% of best	Increased symptoms, nocturnal wakening, increased need for bronchodilator	Start oral corticosteroids. Contact doctor as soon as possible
<40% of best	Severe symptoms, no relief with bronchodilator	Call ambulance. Continue to use bronchodilator

- In a patient with symptoms of asthma but normal spirometry, home peak flow monitoring may establish the diagnosis. Diurnal variability of >15% strongly suggests asthma.
- In *occupational* asthma, peak flows can be very helpful. Characteristic improvements and deteriorations in peak flow values related to time at work and off work over a period of at least 2 weeks can clinch the diagnosis. This evidence can be supported by the demonstration of bronchial hyperresponsiveness (see Chapter 7).

Peak expiratory flow technique

Peak flow is very dependent on patient technique. It is essential that the correct technique is established before home monitoring is undertaken. The patient should:
- stand or sit up straight
- inhale maximally ('breathe in all the way')
- get a good seal around the mouthpiece

- blow out as hard and as fast as possible ('blast out')
- continue to exhale for 1–2 seconds (it is not necessary to prolong expiration as in spirometry)

Three measurements should be obtained (there are no agreed criteria for reproducibility).

By convention the highest of the three measurements is reported (the 'best' of three).

It is important to know if the measurements were done before or after the administration of a bronchodilator.

CHAPTER SUMMARY

→ The peak expiratory flow is very effort-dependent.
→ Peak flows are better for monitoring than for diagnosing airflow obstruction.
→ >15% diurnal variability suggests a diagnosis of asthma.
→ All asthmatics should know what their best peak flow is, as a baseline to assess the severity of future asthma attacks.

. . . see over for clinical examples

Clinical example

Patient 3A: age 15, female, European, height 1.60 m, weight 56 kg

History: Nocturnal dry cough and 'tightness' in the chest. Spirometry normal when seen in clinic.

The patient was asked to keep a morning and evening peak flow diary for 3 weeks (Fig. 3.1).

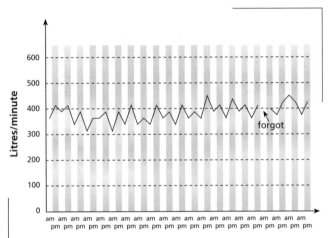

Figure 3.1 Peak expiratory flow diary
This shows diurnal (morning–evening) variability as well as changes in peak expiratory flow from day to day.

Interpretation: The diary shows significant variability in peak flow and diurnal variation (morning–evening peak flow/mean peak flow) of over 15%. Her 'best' peak flow is 450 L/minute. She should try to remember this for future reference, and an interim action plan could be based on this figure. She may achieve higher peak flows when she has been established on treatment and this 'best' peak flow figure will need to be reviewed.

Chapter 4
Lung volumes

More detailed assessment of lung function usually includes the measurement of the static lung volumes. These can be very helpful in sorting out restrictive and obstructive disorders. The most important measurements are:

- *Total lung capacity* (TLC): the volume of air in the thorax at full inspiration—the maximum volume of air that the lungs can contain. This is limited by the mechanics of the chest wall, the respiratory muscles used in inspiration and lung compliance (lung 'stretchiness').

- *Residual volume* (RV): the volume of air left in the thorax at full expiration—the little bit of air that cannot be breathed out. This is determined by chest wall mechanics, the respiratory muscles of expiration, the elastic recoil of the lungs and in some cases (particularly the elderly and those with airways disease) by airways collapse, usually at the lung bases, preventing further air from escaping.

- *Functional residual capacity* (FRC): the volume of air in the thorax when no inspiratory or expiratory effort is being made—what is left after a quiet, unforced expiration. At this volume the outward 'springiness' of the chest wall balances the elastic recoil of the lungs.

The relationship between these measurements is shown in Figure 4.1. Other measurements are sometimes quoted, such as inspiratory reserve volume (IRV) and expiratory reserve volume (ERV) which are simply the differences between FRC plus tidal volume and TLC, and between FRC and RV respectively. Each of the factors determining the lung volumes can be altered by disease.

Measurement of lung volumes requires a method of estimating the volume of gas inside the thorax. There are two basic ways of doing this: helium dilution and the body plethysmograph.

Helium dilution allows the air in the thorax to equilibrate with a known volume of air containing a small concentration of helium. The final dilution of helium is used to calculate the volume of air in the thorax (Fig. 4.2). The body plethysmograph ('body box') uses the small fluctuations in pressure inside a sealed box containing the patient during breathing to calculate the volume of gas in the thorax (for a more detailed explanation see *The body plethysmograph*). It is important to know which of these methods has been used because, although they should give the same results in healthy lungs, the results may differ in some circumstances. For example, the helium dilution technique may underestimate lung volumes in a patient with bullous disease because the helium may not mix with all parts of the lung (Fig. 4.2(c)). In general, the body box is regarded as the more accurate technique, but is more demanding for the patient and more technically complex.

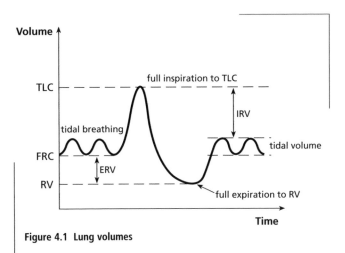

Figure 4.1 Lung volumes

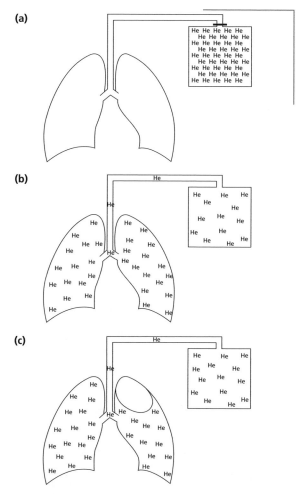

Figure 4.2 Measurement of thoracic gas volume (VTG) using helium dilution

(a) A known volume and concentration of helium is allowed to equilibrate with the air in the lungs. (b) The volume of gas in the thorax can be calculated from the final concentration of helium. (c) A bulla or poorly communicating area of the lung will lead to underestimation of the lung volumes if this does not allow equilibration of helium.

THE BODY PLETHYSMOGRAPH

Although you do not need to know how the plethysmograph (body box) works in order to interpret lung function results, an understanding of the basic principles is useful (and interesting).

The basic principle behind the body box is Boyle's law, which states that for a given mass of gas the product of the pressure and the volume remains constant, providing that the temperature doesn't change:

$$P_1 \times V_1 = P_2 \times V_2$$

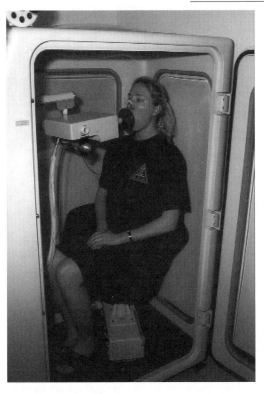

Figure 4.3 A subject in the body plethysmograph (body box)—the door is shut during testing

where P_1 and V_1 are the pressure and volume of a mass of gas and P_2 and V_2 are the pressure and volume of the same mass of gas after a change in pressure and volume. The equation can also be written:

$$P_1 \times V_1 = (P_1 + \Delta P) \times (V_1 + \Delta V)$$

where ΔP is the change in pressure and ΔV is the associated change in volume.

To measure lung volumes, the patient sits inside the sealed body box. Inside the box there are two masses of gas: one in the thorax, and one outside the body. The volume of the gas outside the body is equal to the volume of the box minus the volume displaced by the patient (which can be estimated from the patient's weight). The pressure inside the box is measured, then a small, known volume of air is introduced into the sealed box to calibrate the pressure change associated with the known volume change.

The patient is asked to take rapid shallow breaths (pant) through a mouthpiece. During this manoeuvre a shutter is closed in the mouthpiece but the patient continues the panting effort. While the shutter is closed, the gas in the lungs does not communicate with gas in the rest of the box. As the patient continues to pant there are fluctuations in the box pressure, due to changes in the volume of gas displaced by the patient as the air in the lungs is alternately compressed and allowed to expand with the respiratory cycle. This volume fluctuation (ΔV) can be calculated from the pressure change. At the same time a pressure transducer inside the mouthpiece records the pressure changes within the mouth. Since the mouth air is in communication with the air in the lung (the patient is instructed to pant against the mouthpiece) and since there is no airflow because the shutter is closed, the mouth pressure equals the pressure in the lung. We now know P_1, P_2 (the two lung pressures as the patient pants in and out against the mouthpiece) and the difference between V_1 and V_2 (ΔV). V_2 can be replaced by ($V_1 + \Delta V$) in Boyle's law and the equation can be solved for V_1.

In practice the volume fluctuations of the lung and the associated pressure changes are measured and plotted against each other to form a diagonal line ($\Delta P/\Delta V$). The *slope* of this line depends on the starting lung volume, and can be used to calculate the volume of the thoracic gas (VTG) by computer.

The VTG is measured close to the FRC. Measuring airflow through the mouthpiece during tidal breathing, maximal inspiration (to TLC) and maximal expiration (to RV) followed by the measurement of VTG in a combined procedure allows the lung volumes to be calculated. The procedure is repeated several times until reproducible results are obtained.

It should be obvious that this technique relies on the accurate measurement of small pressure changes. Calibration of the instruments and correction for temperature changes within the box during the procedure should minimise errors, but the possibility of small inaccuracies leading to large errors in the results should be borne in mind.

Total lung capacity and residual volume

In obstructive lung diseases, the narrowing and closure of airways during expiration tends to lead to 'gas trapping' within the lungs and 'hyperinflation' of the chest. Gas trapping leads to an increase in RV while hyperinflation increases the TLC (Fig. 4.4). Although both values increase, the RV tends to have a greater percentage increase than TLC. The RV/TLC ratio is therefore also increased. Sometimes gas trapping occurs (raised RV) without hyperinflation.

In restrictive disorders the cardinal feature is a reduction in TLC. Be cautious about diagnosing a restrictive disorder if the TLC is normal—a high FEV_1/FVC ratio with a normal TLC is more likely to be due to poorly performed spirometry than to true restriction. In fibrotic lung disease the RV also falls because of increased elastic recoil (stiffness) of the lungs and loss of alveoli (Fig. 4.5). Chest wall disease (such as neuromuscular disease or kyphoscoliosis) can also cause a restrictive pattern in which the TLC is reduced—either because of mechanical limitation to chest wall expansion or because of respiratory muscle weakness. Nevertheless, the lung tissue (and therefore the elastic recoil) is normal and the RV tends to be preserved, leading to a high RV/TLC ratio.

In some patients there may be a *mixed pattern* of restrictive and obstructive disorders. This may occur because a single disease (for example, sarcoidosis) affects both the lung parenchyma and the airways or because of the coexistence of two common diseases such as chronic obstructive pulmonary disease and fibrosing alveolitis. This may be indicated by an obstructive pattern on spirometry or flow-volume loop, combined with reduced lung volumes.

Lung volumes are also useful when there are equivocal findings on spirometry. For example if the FEV_1 and FVC are at the lower limit of normal, the finding of a raised TLC or RV supports a diagnosis of obstruction. Conversely, if the spirometric values and lung volumes are

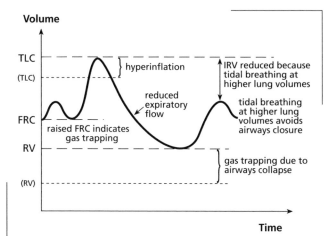

Figure 4.4 Changes in lung volumes in obstructive disorders
(volumes in parentheses are the predicted TLC and RV)

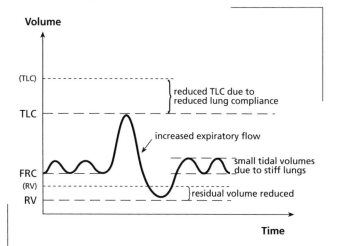

Figure 4.5 Changes in lung volumes in restrictive disorders
(volumes in parentheses are the predicted TLC and RV)

all mildly reduced (or increased) by a similar amount the patient probably has normal but slightly smaller (or bigger) than average lungs.

Functional residual capacity

Different respiratory diseases may alter the volume of air in the lungs during tidal breathing; this is measured by the FRC. Gas trapping and airways closure at low lung volumes cause patients with obstructive disorders, particularly emphysema, to breathe at high lung volumes. This has the benefit of preventing airways closure and improves ventilation-perfusion relationships, but reduces the mechanical advantage of the respiratory muscles and increases the work of breathing (try breathing at a high FRC yourself and feel what it is like).

In restrictive disorders due to lung fibrosis, breathing takes place at a low FRC because of the increased effort needed to expand the lungs. This reduces the work of breathing but leads to atelectasis (small areas of lung collapse) which reduces ventilation-perfusion ratios and makes the lungs stiffer (lower compliance). Obesity may also cause patients to breathe at a low FRC because of the weight of the chest wall and compromised movement of the diaphragm.

The FRC is normally reduced when a person is lying down because gravity no longer helps by pulling the abdominal contents away from the thorax. This may reduce gas exchange in obese patients or patients with lung disease. However, the FRC is rarely, if ever, measured lying down.

The inspiratory and expiratory reserve volumes (IRV and ERV) are simply calculated from the FRC, TLC and RV and add little to the interpretation of them.

CHAPTER SUMMARY

→ Measurement of lung volumes is a useful adjunct to spirometry to help distinguish between obstructive and restrictive disorders.

→ Obstructive disorders increase the RV and TLC. The RV/TLC ratio tends to be high.

→ Restrictive disorders reduce the TLC. The RV is also reduced in lung fibrosis.

Clinical examples

Patient 4A: age 68, male, European, height 1.78 m, weight 83 kg

History: Gradual onset of dyspnoea and cough.

Technician's comments: good patient technique, results acceptable and reproducible.

		Predicted	Measured	% predicted
Spirometry	FEV_1 litres	3.00	2.14	71
	FVC litres	4.42	(2.82)	(64)
	FEV_1/FVC %	69	76	
	$FEF_{25-75\%}$ L/s	2.74	1.65	60

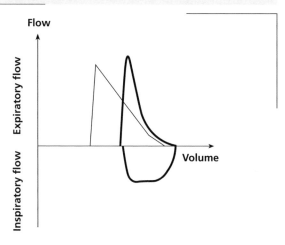

Figure 4.6

This flow-volume loop was performed in the body plethysmograph at the same time as measurement of lung volumes. This means that the lung volumes at the start and end of the loop (TLC and RV) are known and the loop can be compared to the shape and position of the predicted loop (thin line). The measured flow-volume loop is shifted to the right, indicating a reduction in lung volumes. It is also narrower than predicted, indicating a reduced vital capacity.

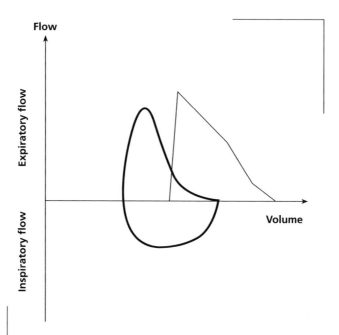

Figure 4.7
This flow-volume loop was also measured in the body plethysmograph at the same time as measurement of lung volumes. This time the measured loop is to the left of the predicted loop, indicating increased TLC and RV.

		Predicted	Measured	% predicted
Lung volumes	TLC litres	5.47	(6.89)	(126)
(plethysmograph)	RV litres	2.12	(3.98)	(187)
	RV/TLC %	39	(58)	
	FRC litres	2.70	4.22	(157)
	VC litres	3.32	2.91	88

Interpretation: Spirometry is within normal limits except for a reduction in mid-expiratory flow. However, the FVC might have been underestimated because the patient was unable to exhale fully. The FEV_1/FVC ratio may therefore be overestimated.

Lung volumes suggest an obstructive pattern with a hyperinflation (raised TLC) and gas trapping (raised RV). The RV/TLC ratio is high and the patient has a high FRC as is typical for obstructive disorders. However, these findings need to be interpreted with caution in view of the technician's comments. There may be significant errors in the plethysmograph measurements because of difficulty with the patient's technique. The patient's chest pain should be investigated and it may be worth repeating the tests when this is better.

Patient 4C: age 60, male, European, height 1.83 m, weight 89 kg

History: Gradual onset of dyspnoea and cough. Ex-smoker.
Technician's comments: good patient technique, results acceptable and reproducible.

		Predicted	Measured	% predicted
Spirometry	FEV$_1$ litres	3.44	(1.18)	(34)
	FVC litres	4.91	(3.29)	(67)
	FEV$_1$/FVC %	70	36	
Lung volumes	TLC litres	7.14	(12.44)	(174)
(plethysmograph)	RV litres	2.51	(9.12)	(364)
	RV/TLC %	37	(73)	
	FRC litres	3.94	(9.76)	(248)
	VC litres	4.91	(3.31)	(67)

The tests were repeated 15 minutes after administration of nebulised bronchodilator.

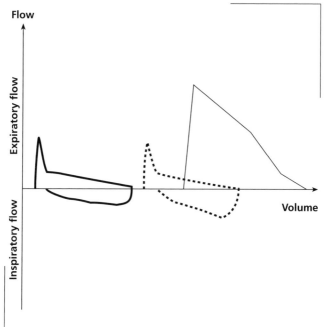

Figure 4.8
The flow-volume loop after bronchodilator is indicated by the broken line.

		Measured	% predicted	% change
Spirometry	FEV$_1$ litres	(1.16)	(34)	−2
	FVC litres	(3.38)	(69)	3
	FEV$_1$/FVC %	34		
Lung volumes	TLC litres	(8.56)	(120)	−31
(plethysmograph)	RV litres	(5.18)	(206)	−43
	RV/TLC %	(61)		
	FRC litres	(5.96)	(151)	−39
	VC litres	(3.38)	(69)	2

Interpretation: There is an obstructive defect with massive hyperinflation and gas trapping. Although there appears to be no response to bronchodilator on spirometry, there is significant improvement of the hyperinflation and gas trapping. This occurs occasionally in chronic obstructive pulmonary disease and emphasises the point that a failure to demonstrate a significant reduction in airflow obstruction does not necessarily mean that the patient will not get symptomatic benefit from a bronchodilator.

Chapter 5

Gas transfer

The primary function of the lungs is to exchange gases. There are two principal processes involved—the exchange of gas between the blood and the alveoli, and the ventilation of the alveoli with air. Carbon dioxide (CO_2) is very soluble in water and moves rapidly across alveolar membranes so that the pressure of carbon dioxide in the alveoli is virtually identical with that in the blood. The rate-limiting step in expiring carbon dioxide is the ventilation of the lung with atmospheric air (which contains virtually no CO_2). For oxygen, which is poorly soluble in water, the diffusion across the alveolar membrane is much slower and so oxygen uptake is more sensitive to alveolar disease than is carbon dioxide removal. Although ventilation is also important for replenishing alveolar oxygen supplies, the rate-limiting step in oxygen exchange is usually exchange across the alveolar membrane. Tests of gas transfer are estimates of the ability of the lungs to take up oxygen.

Diffusing capacity (DL$_{CO}$)

The diffusing capacity of the lungs is estimated using carbon monoxide (CO). CO has similar physical properties to oxygen in terms of its solubility and ability to diffuse across membranes. It also has the advantage of being very strongly bound to haemoglobin, so that all the CO transferred across the alveolar wall is retained within the circulation and not exhaled. There are numerous protocols for performing the test but all involve inhaling a small, known quantity of carbon monoxide and comparing this with the concentration of carbon monoxide in the exhaled air. An inert gas (helium, methane or neon) is used to distinguish between the dilution of carbon monoxide with the air in the lungs and the uptake of carbon monoxide into the blood (see *Measurement of gas transfer*). The term 'diffusing capacity' is somewhat misleading because the test is less dependent on the diffusion of carbon monoxide than on the matching of alveolar ventilation with pulmonary blood flow (see below). It is also dependent on the binding of carbon monoxide to haemoglobin. For these reasons the term 'transfer factor' (TL$_{CO}$) is sometimes preferred.

MEASUREMENT OF GAS TRANSFER

There are several techniques for measuring the DL$_{CO}$. They can be divided into single breath (the most common) and steady state methods. All the methods are based on the principles of Fick's law of diffusion. This states that the diffusion of a gas across a membrane is proportional to the area of membrane, the pressure of the gas across the membrane and the diffusing constant of the gas, and inversely proportional to the thickness of the membrane. When measuring the diffusing capacity of the lungs (in which the area/thickness of the membranes is part of what we want to measure) this simplifies to:

$$\dot{V}_{CO} = DL_{CO} \times PA_{CO}$$

where $\dot{V}_{CO}$ = rate of uptake of CO

PA$_{CO}$ = alveolar pressure of CO (the CO pressure of the blood is assumed to be zero)

or:

$$DL_{CO} = \dot{V}_{CO}/PA_{CO}$$

The various techniques differ in how they measure PA$_{CO}$ and $\dot{V}_{CO}$. Only the single breath-hold technique is described here.

A single breath is taken from RV to TLC of a gas mixture containing a known (small) concentration of carbon monoxide and a known concentration of an inert gas (helium or methane) plus 21% oxygen. The breath is held at TLC for 10 seconds (time T). During exhalation the first part of the exhaled air is discarded to allow for anatomical dead space (the gas in the upper airway, trachea and bronchi that does not participate in gas exchange). A sample of gas is taken from mid-exhalation and analysed. This is assumed to be representative of alveolar gas.

The initial alveolar pressure of CO depends on the inhaled concentration of CO and the dilution by gases already in the airway. This dilution can be calculated by measuring the inert gas on exhalation, because this is not taken up by the lung and its final concentration is the same as at the start of the breath-hold. Thus:

$$\text{initial alveolar concentration of CO} = \text{Fico} \times \text{FAHe}/\text{FiHe}$$

where   Fico   = fraction of CO in inspired gas

       FiHe   = fraction of helium (or methane) in inspired gas

       FAHe   = fraction of helium (or methane) in exhaled alveolar sample

The alveolar volume (VA) can also be calculated with the inert gas using the principles of the He dilution technique (Chapter 3).

Thus the initial (FA_{CO_0}) and final (FA_{CO_T}) alveolar concentrations of CO are known. The concentration of CO will have decreased exponentially in the time between the measurements of these two and the rate of uptake of CO ($\dot{V}_{CO}$) is calculated from the natural logarithm (ln) of the ratio of the FA_{CO_0}/FA_{CO_T}.

The DLco can be calculated:

$$DL_{CO} = \frac{VA}{T \times (PB - 47)} \times \ln \frac{FA_{CO_0}}{FA_{CO_T}}$$

where   T = time of breath-hold

           PB = barometric pressure

           47 = water vapour pressure at 37°C

To calculate the Kco (DLco/VA) the equation is simply:

$$K_{CO} = \frac{1}{T \times (PB - 47)} \times \ln \frac{FA_{CO_0}}{FA_{CO_T}}$$

Although the diffusion of oxygen (and therefore carbon monoxide) across the alveolar wall is much slower than that of carbon dioxide, in normal lungs the full saturation of haemoglobin is usually achieved in one-third of the time that the red blood cell is in the alveolar capillary. This means that a very large impediment to diffusion is necessary before there is any significant effect on gas transfer. In practice, thickening of the alveolar wall usually has little effect on the DLco. Far more important is mismatch of ventilation and perfusion ($\dot{V}/\dot{Q}$ mismatch). This means that ventilation to parts of the lung that have little or no pulmonary blood supply is wasted and that some of the pulmonary circulation passes through the lungs without coming into contact with functioning alveoli.

The DL_{CO} is reduced in any disease that allows blood to pass through poorly ventilated areas of lung. Acutely this includes pneumonic consolidation, collapse (due to bronchial obstruction or atelectasis from poor lung expansion) and adult respiratory distress syndrome (ARDS), in which extensive areas of the lungs are oedematous. It is also reduced in conditions such as pulmonary embolism which permit ventilation to areas of the lung without adequate perfusion (see *Disorders associated with a reduced DL_{CO}*).

DISORDERS ASSOCIATED WITH A REDUCED DL_{CO}

Disorders associated with a reduced DL_{CO} include:

- *diseases of the pulmonary circulation*
    - pulmonary thromboembolic disease
    - idiopathic pulmonary arterial hypertension
    - arteriovenous malformations
    - vasculitis (for example, scleroderma, SLE)
- *conditions affecting alveoli*
    - pneumonic consolidation or areas of lung collapse
    - emphysema
    - ARDS
    - fibrotic lung diseases (for example, cryptogenic fibrosing alveolitis, drug-induced fibrosis, asbestosis)
    - granulomatous diseases (for example, hypersensitivity pneumonitis, sarcoidosis)
    - lung resection
- *cardiac diseases*
    - pulmonary oedema
    - right-left shunt (congenital cyanotic heart disease or Eisenmenger's syndrome)
- *miscellaneous conditions*
    - anaemia
    - pregnancy (approximately 15% decrease, mechanism uncertain)
    - recent smoking (high carbon monoxide tension in blood reduces uptake)

Destructive lung disorders such as emphysema reduce gas transfer because of wasted ventilation to areas of the lung with few effective alveoli (such as bullae) and because the pulmonary circulation is also forced to bypass effective alveoli. Interstitial lung diseases, such as fibrosing alveolitis, also reduce the DLco because part of the pulmonary circulation passes through areas of lung with destroyed alveoli.

The DLco may be increased in conditions that increase the amount of haemoglobin available to bind carbon monoxide. In effect, this includes conditions in which pulmonary blood volume is increased (left-to-right shunt, exercise, supine position), poly-cythaemia and pulmonary haemorrhage syndromes (such as Goodpasture's syndrome). Two conditions in which a raised DLco is occasionally seen are asthma and massive obesity. The mechanisms behind these are uncertain.

CORRECTION OF THE DLco FOR HAEMOGLOBIN

Many lung function laboratories will automatically correct the DLco if the haemoglobin is provided. The most widely used equations are based on J. E. Cotes, J. M. Dabbs, P. C. Elwood, A. M. Hall, A. MacDonald & M. J. Saunders, 'Iron deficiency anaemia: its effect on transfer factor for the lung (diffusing capacity) and ventilation and cardiac frequency during submaximal exercise', *Clin Sci* 1972, 42, pp. 325–35.

MEN (ADJUSTS THE DLco TO A HAEMOGLOBIN OF 14.6 g/dL)

$$\text{Hb-adjusted DLco} = \text{Observed DLco} \times \frac{(10.22 + \text{Hb})}{1.7 \times \text{Hb}}$$

WOMEN AND CHILDREN UNDER 15 YEARS (ADJUSTS THE DLco TO A HAEMOGLOBIN OF 13.4 g/dL)

$$\text{Hb-adjusted DLco} = \text{Observed DLco} \times \frac{(9.38 + \text{Hb})}{1.7 \times \text{Hb}}$$

These adjustments are based on a theoretical approach which does not take into account the possibility of a physiological compensation for the haemoglobin level. For example, in severe anaemia there may be an increase in cardiac output which would increase the pulmonary blood volume. This would increase the DLco and the above equations may be an overadjustment.

In anaemia and polycythaemia the DLco can be corrected for the level of haemoglobin if this is known. Most pulmonary function laboratories will do this if provided with the haemoglobin (see *Correction of the DLco for haemoglobin*). A (very) approximate adjustment is to reduce the predicted value by 4% for each g/dL below normal haemoglobin (14.6 for men, 13.4 for women and children), and increase it by 2% for each g/dL above normal. The haemoglobin or haematocrit should be checked if the DLco is abnormal or if the DLco changes during follow-up of a patient.

Recent cigarette smoking (or exposure to other sources of environmental carbon monoxide) will reduce the DLco by about 1% for each 1% increase in carboxyhaemoglobin. This has the effect of reducing the haemoglobin available for the binding of further CO (an 'anaemia' effect), and creating a 'back pressure' of CO in exhaled air, reducing the apparent uptake of CO during the test. This effect should be avoided by asking the patient not to smoke on the day of the test. Alternatively, the blood level of carboxyhaemoglobin can be measured and the DLco value adjusted for this blood level.

The DLco is a sensitive test for many lung diseases. In interstitial lung disease (for example, fibrosing alveolitis) in particular it may be reduced before abnormalities in other pulmonary function tests become apparent. This should always be considered if there is an isolated reduction in DLco without an obvious cause (such as anaemia).

Krogh constant (Kco, DLco/VA)

The Krogh constant (Kco or DLco/VA) is an attempt to adjust the DLco for differences in lung volume. The alveolar volume (VA) is estimated by the inhalation of an inert gas at the same time as carbon monoxide in the same way as in the helium dilution technique (see above). The Kco is calculated by dividing the DLco by the VA and is often (more correctly) denoted DLco/VA. Differences in DLco due to the size of the patient's lungs are 'corrected' by the Kco. For example, smaller patients have lower carbon monoxide uptake because the alveolar area available for gas transfer is less, but the Kco should be the same as in larger patients. In patients who have had lung resection the DLco is reduced because of loss of alveoli. Providing the remaining lung tissue is normal the Kco should be normal (in fact it may be increased because of the increased pulmonary blood flow to the remaining lung). It follows that when the K_{CO} does not correct to normal there is likely to be an abnormality of the lung tissue.

It does not follow that a normal K_{CO} implies normal gas transfer. For example, areas of poorly ventilated lung will reduce the DL_{CO}, but will also reduce the VA because of the poor distribution of helium, and the DL_{CO}/VA may be normal. In restrictive lung diseases such as fibrosing alveolitis, the destruction of alveolar tissue may lead to a profound reduction in gas transfer. However, this will be underestimated by the DL_{CO}/VA because the reduction in lung volume also reduces the VA. For this reason the K_{CO} should only be interpreted in the context of the DL_{CO}.

The VA (estimated by the helium dilution technique) should be similar to the TLC measured in the body box. A big difference between these measures is a clue to the presence of uneven distribution of ventilation such as in bullous emphysema.

CHAPTER SUMMARY

→ The DL_{CO} is a sensitive measure of pulmonary gas exchange.
→ The DL_{CO}/VA or K_{CO} is useful to distinguish between intrinsic lung disease and loss of lung tissue.
→ The DL_{CO} needs to be corrected for the haemoglobin level.

. . . see over for clinical examples

Clinical examples

Patient 5A: age 56, male, European, height 1.84 m, weight 82 kg

History: Progressive dyspnoea. Heavy smoker in past.

Technician's comments: Technique satisfactory. Patient had his bronchodilator 2 hours before the test.

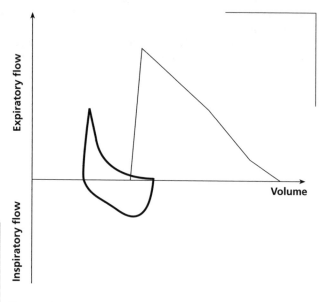

Figure 5.1

		Predicted	Measured	% predicted
Spirometry	FEV$_1$ litres	3.57	(1.12)	(31)
	FVC litres	5.01	(2.14)	(43)
	FEV$_1$/FVC %	71	52	
	FEF$_{25-75\%}$ L/s	3.38	(0.50)	(15)

Lung volumes	TLC litres	7.20	(9.67)	(134)
(plethysmograph)	RV litres	2.44	(6.35)	(260)
	RV/TLC %	36	(66)	
	FRC litres	4.03	(7.11)	(176)
	VC litres	5.01	(3.33)	(66)
Gas transfer				
	DLco mL/min/mmHg	25.4	(14.5)	(57)
	DLco/VA mL/min/mmHg/L	3.92	4.04	103
	VA litres		3.59	

Interpretation: Spirometry shows a severe obstructive defect. Lung volumes show hyperinflation, gas trapping and a high RV/TLC ratio. The DLco is low, consistent with emphysema (haemoglobin was normal). The DLco appears to correct for alveolar volume: the DLco/VA is normal, but this is because the VA is underestimated (it should be similar to the TLC), indicating that there are large, poorly ventilated areas of the lung—probably emphysematous bullae. Note that the unforced vital capacity (VC) is greater than the FVC—this suggests airways collapse during the forced manoeuvre.

Patient 5B: age 24, female, European, height 1.72 m, weight 50 kg

History: Intermittent dyspnoea and wheeze. Non-smoker.
Technician's comments: Technique satisfactory, results acceptable and reproducible.

		Predicted	Measured	% predicted
Spirometry	FEV₁ litres	3.52	(1.74)	(49)
	FVC litres	4.39	(3.17)	(72)
	FEV₁/FVC%	80	55	
	FEF₂₅₋₇₅% L/s	3.91	(0.65)	(17)

Lung volumes	TLC litres	5.99	5.92	99
(plethysmograph)	RV litres	1.84	(2.62)	(142)
	RV/TLC %	28	(44)	
	FRC litres	3.59	3.79	105
	VC litres	4.39	(3.30)	(75)
Gas transfer				
	DLco mL/min/mmHg	22.2	(26.2)	(118)
	DLco/VA mL/min/mmHg/L	4.80	5.95	124
	VA litres		4.39	

Spirometry was repeated 15 minutes after nebulised bronchodilator:

	Measured	% predicted	% change
FEV_1 litres	(2.80)	(80)	61
FVC litres	(3.21)	(73)	1
FEV_1/FVC %	87		
$FEF_{25-75\%}$ L/s	(3.04)	(78)	366

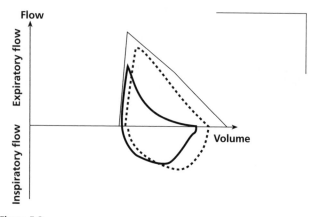

Figure 5.2
The flow-volume loop after bronchodilator is indicated by the broken line.

Interpretation: Spirometry shows a moderately severe obstructive defect. There was a significant response to bronchodilator. Lung volumes show gas trapping but not hyperinflation. The DLco is near the upper limit of normal, consistent with asthma. The VA is lower than the TLC, indicating that there are large poorly ventilated areas of the lung. Note that the unforced vital capacity (VC) is similar to the FVC—there is little airways collapse during the forced manoeuvre.

Patient 5C: age 77, male, European, height 1.64 m, weight 73 kg

History: Gradual onset of dyspnoea and cough over the past few months. Smoked approximately 20 cigarettes a day for 30 years, but gave up smoking 15 years ago. Has been treated with amiodarone for atrial fibrillation. Has a pet parrot.

Technician's comments: Good patient technique, but coughed when trying to expire fully. FVC may be underestimated.

		Predicted	Measured	% predicted
Spirometry	FEV$_1$ litres	2.26	2.08	92
	FVC litres	3.45	2.55	74
	FEV$_1$/FVC %	68	81	
	FEF$_{25-75\%}$ L/s	2.10	2.09	99
Lung volumes	TLC litres	5.21	(3.81)	(73)
(plethysmograph)	RV litres	2.32	(1.26)	(54)
	RV/TLC %	43	33	
	FRC litres	3.07	2.03	66
	VC litres	3.45	2.55	74
Gas transfer				
	DLco mL/min/mmHg	16.3	(5.9)	(36)
	DLco/VA mL/min/mmHg/L	3.45	1.83	53
	VA litres		3.23	

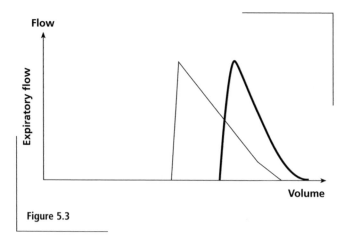

Figure 5.3

Interpretation: (This is the same patient as Patient 1D in Chapter 1.)
Lung volumes and gas transfer have now been added to spirometry.
The lung volumes confirm the restrictive pattern suggested by the
low/normal FVC and high FEV_1/FVC ratio. Gas transfer is severely
reduced. This is compatible with interstitial lung disease—either
amiodarone lung or extrinsic allergic alveolitis (due to exposure
to birds) could give this pattern, as could any other form of lung
fibrosis.

Chapter 6
Respiratory muscle function

R espiratory muscle strength can be tested by measuring the pressure generated by inspiring and expiring against a closed airway. Healthy adults can generate a *maximal inspiratory pressure* (MIP) of greater than –60 cmH$_2$O, and a *maximal expiratory pressure* (MEP) of greater than 80 cmH$_2$O (both pressures tend to be higher in males and decline with age). Pressures lower than these may indicate neuromuscular disease affecting the muscles of respiration. However, other disorders may reduce the pressures by placing the respiratory muscles at a mechanical disadvantage. For example, the pressures may be reduced if there is chest wall deformity. MIPs may be reduced by hyperinflation/gas trapping which flattens the diaphragm and places the intercostal muscles at a disadvantage. MEPs may also be reduced in severe obstructive lung diseases. A MEP of less than 40 cmH$_2$O leads to an ineffective cough.

MIPs/MEPs are useful in the assessment of respiratory failure. They are sometimes used to predict whether a patient can be weaned from a ventilator. They are occasionally helpful in the diagnosis of unexplained breathlessness in association with a low vital capacity. However, their usefulness is limited by the wide range of normal values and the fact that the tests are very effort-dependent. MIPs and MEPs are hard to perform and require a highly motivated subject.

Measuring the FVC while erect and supine can be used to detect diaphragmatic weakness. If this is present, the supine FVC is lower, because the effect of gravity in keeping the abdominal contents out of the thorax is lost.

More sophisticated tests of respiratory muscle function are available. For example transdiaphragmatic pressures can be measured using gastric and oesophageal balloons. However, these are not often used clinically. For a comprehensive review of respiratory muscle testing, see 'ATS/ERS statement on respiratory muscle testing', *American Journal of Respiratory and Critical Care Medicine*, 2002, 166, pp. 518–624 (also available from the ATS website—see the bibliography at the back of the book).

CHAPTER SUMMARY

➔ MIPs and MEPs are useful in assessing respiratory failure due to neuromuscular disease.

➔ They are occasionally useful in patients with unexplained dyspnoea.

➔ The range of 'normal values' is wide.

➔ Measurement of MIPs and MEPs is very dependent on patient effort.

Clinical example

Patient 6A: age 51, male, European, height 1.69 m, weight 85.8 kg

History: Progressive muscle weakness. Presents with type II (ventilatory) respiratory failure and polycythaemia. Non-smoker.

Technician's comments: Good patient technique, results reproducible.

		Predicted	Measured	% predicted
Spirometry	FEV$_1$ litres	3.63	(1.40)	(39)
	FVC litres	4.57	(1.60)	(35)
	FEV$_1$/FVC %	79	84	
Lung volumes	TLC litres	6.43	(3.24)	(50)
(plethysmograph)	RV litres	2.04	1.56	77
	RV/TLC %	30	(48)	
	FRC litres	2.98	(1.74)	(58)
	VC litres	4.57	(1.68)	(37)
Gas transfer				
DLco mL/min/mmHg		32.8	(20.6)	(63)
DLco/VA mL/min/mmHg/L		5.38	8.32	154
VA litres		6.10	2.48	
Maximal pressures	MIP cmH$_2$O	<−60	(−33)	
	MEP cmH$_2$O	>80	(33)	

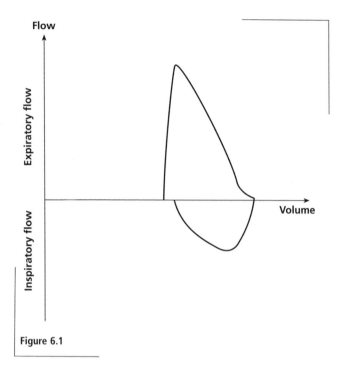

Figure 6.1

Interpretation: Spirometry and lung volumes suggest a restrictive defect. The RV is relatively preserved and there is a high RV/TLC ratio. Gas transfer is impaired but corrects for alveolar volume (the DLco values have been adjusted for the raised haemoglobin). The history suggests that the restrictive defect could be due to respiratory muscle weakness and this is confirmed by the reduced MIPs and MEPs. The patient was treated with non-invasive ventilation. The diagnosis was myotonic dystrophy. (The FRC in this patient was reduced—the FRC is often normal in patients with restriction due to respiratory muscle weakness.)

Chapter 7

Bronchial challenge

Asthma is characterised by variable airflow obstruction. This variability is partly due to hyperreactivity of airway smooth muscle, leading to bronchoconstriction in response to certain stimuli. This can be tested in the respiratory laboratory by measuring the change in lung function following exposure to stimuli. These tests are particularly useful if the history suggests episodic asthma, but there is no convincing evidence of airway obstruction at the time the patient is assessed.

There are numerous protocols and challenge agents in use. Most measure the fall in FEV_1 in response to increasing exposure to an inhaled chemical. For safety reasons, bronchial challenge is not generally recommended if the initial FEV_1 is less than 65% predicted. Recent use of bronchodilating drugs or antihistamines may make the test falsely negative and should be avoided. A recent respiratory tract infection may cause a false positive test.

Chemical stimuli

Methacholine and histamine are commonly used bronchial challenge agents. They are regarded as *direct* stimuli because they act directly on airway smooth muscle, causing bronchospasm. They are usually administered in increasing concentrations from a nebuliser at intervals of 1–3 minutes, and followed by measurement of the FEV_1. The results are often quoted as the provocative concentration or dose

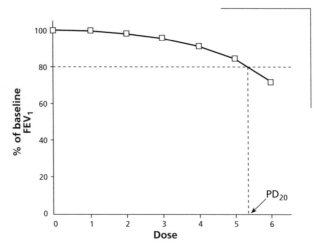

Figure 7.1 Bronchial challenge
Increasing doses of the challenge agent (for example, methacholine) are
administered until a 20% fall in FEV_1 is achieved. The dose required to produce a
20% fall (PD_{20}) can be calculated from the dose-response curve.

required to produce a 20% fall in FEV_1 (PC_{20} or PD_{20}) (Fig. 7.1). The
lower the PC_{20} or PD_{20}, the worse the bronchial hyperresponsiveness.
A PC_{20} of less than 8 mg/mL or a PD_{20} of less than 8 µmol are often
regarded as positive but this may vary according to the protocol used.

A number of *indirect* stimuli are now in use. These do not act on
airway smooth muscle causing constriction directly but through a
number of intermediate steps, such as causing histamine release from
mast cells or by stimulation of airway nerves. The relative merits of
these agents over histamine or methacholine are controversial but it
has been suggested that they may more accurately reflect airway
inflammation and may be better for monitoring the response to
anti-inflammatory treatment. Hypertonic saline (and other *osmotic*
challenge agents such as mannitol) is thought to work by altering the
osmolarity of the fluid lining the airways. The effect of this appears to
be similar to the airway-drying effect of exercise. Hence hypertonic
saline is an alternative to exercise or eucapnic hyperventilation
challenges (see below). Hypertonic saline may also have a particular

role in testing for bronchial hyperresponsiveness in SCUBA divers (since divers may inhale salty water during a dive and an asthma attack underwater may be fatal).

Allergen challenge may be useful in determining a likely cause of asthma symptoms, especially in the investigation of suspected occupational asthma. This can be done either in a dose–response manner using allergen extracts, or simply by exposing the patient to an allergen source (such as a cat or wood dust). Allergen challenges are tests of *specific* bronchial hyperresponsiveness because they test a possible aetiological agent of asthma. They are performed much less often than *non-specific* challenges using agents such as methacholine, histamine or hypertonic saline. Allergen challenge should be performed only by experienced persons because of the significant risks associated with them.

Physical stimuli

Spirometry before and after vigorous exercise may be useful in confirming exercise-induced asthma in patients with normal resting lung function. The fall in FEV_1 usually occurs in the first 5–10 minutes after the exercise stops, rather than during exercise. The mechanism is thought to be bronchospasm due to cooling and drying of the airways, and the sensitivity of the test can be increased by the patient inhaling dry or cold air during the exercise. A fall in FEV_1 of 15–20% is significant. *Eucapnic hyperventilation* probably works by a similar mechanism of cooling and drying the airways. In this test hyperventilation of room temperature or cold air is sustained for several minutes. CO_2 is added to the inspired air to prevent respiratory alkalosis. Spirometry is tested at intervals for 20 minutes after hyperventilation ceases. Again, a fall of 15–20% in FEV_1 is significant.

Interpreting bronchial responsiveness

In general, the level of bronchial responsiveness reflects the underlying severity of the asthma. However, the nature of the relationship between bronchial hyperresponsiveness and airway disease is uncertain. It is well recognised that normal individuals with no evidence of asthma may have a positive response to challenge testing. Equally, some patients with unequivocal asthma may have a negative response. This may particularly occur if they have been treated with inhaled corticosteroid. However, changes in PC_{20} or PD_{20} are not reliable ways of assessing response to treatment in individuals. Bronchial challenge tests are not useful for distinguishing between asthma and chronic obstructive pulmonary disease (COPD) because patients with COPD can also show bronchial hyperresponsiveness, although this is less consistent than in asthma.

CHAPTER SUMMARY

→ Tests of bronchial hyperresponsiveness can be *direct* (histamine/methacholine) or *indirect* (hypertonic saline) and *specific* (allergen/exercise) or *non-specific* (methacholine/saline).

→ Most (but not all) asthmatics have bronchial hyperresponsiveness to non-specific stimuli.

→ Most non-asthmatics do not have bronchial hyperresponsiveness.

→ Recent treatment with bronchodilators or antihistamines may lead to a false-negative result.

Clinical example

Patient 7A: age 29, female, European, height 1.67 m, weight 69.1 kg

History: Intermittent dyspnoea on exertion, dry cough.

Technician's comments: Good patient technique, results reproducible.

		Predicted	Measured	% predicted
Spirometry	FEV$_1$ litres	3.33	3.80	114
	FVC litres	3.96	4.93	124
	FEV$_1$/FVC %	84	77	
Lung volumes	TLC litres	5.33	6.34	119
(plethysmograph)	RV litres	1.46	1.41	97
	RV/TLC %	27	22	
	FRC litres	2.70	3.00	111
	VC litres	3.96	4.93	124

Methacholine challenge   PD$_{20}$ (µmol)   1.59

(Severe bronchial hyperresponsiveness PD$_{20}$ < 0.1; moderate 0.1–1.2; mild 1.2–8)

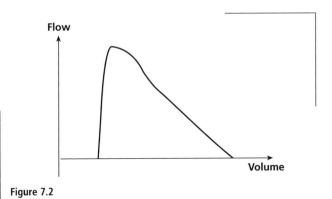

Figure 7.2

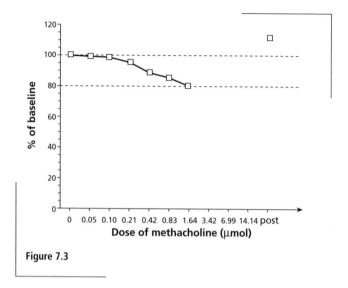

Figure 7.3

Interpretation: Spirometry and lung volumes are at the upper limit of normal. The expiratory flow-volume loop is probably normal, although there is a hint of obstruction. The methacholine challenge demonstrates mild bronchial hyperresponsiveness ($PD_{20} = 1.59$ µmol) which is consistent with a diagnosis of asthma. Note that the 'post'-FEV_1 (after the effects of methacholine were reversed with salbutamol) is about 10% higher than the starting FEV_1.

Chapter 8
Arterial blood gas analysis

Arterial blood gas analysis is the most basic test of the overall capacity of the respiratory system to exchange carbon dioxide for oxygen (see *Obtaining arterial blood gas samples*). It is also used to assess acid–base balance. Blood gas analysers measure the pressure (or tension) of oxygen (P_{O_2}) and carbon dioxide (P_{CO_2}) in the sample and also measure pH. These measurements are often used to provide a number of calculated values. It is easiest to look at the Pa_{CO_2} and pH first.

OBTAINING ARTERIAL BLOOD GAS SAMPLES

Arterial samples are usually obtained from the radial, brachial or femoral artery using a heparinised syringe. Care must be taken not to damage the artery. If the radial artery is used, it is advisable to check for the presence of an ulnar pulse or use the modified Allen's test (where pressure is applied over the ulnar and radial arteries while the patient clenches a fist. When the patient opens the fist, the hand remains ischaemic. Releasing the pressure over the ulnar artery leads to a prompt blush over the hand if the artery is patent). An alternative is to use a capillary sample—often from the ear-lobe (or a heel prick in infants). This requires that the ear lobe is carefully 'arterialised' first, using warmth and sometimes topical vasodilators such as nitroglycerin. Samples should be analysed within a few minutes, or kept on ice if there is likely to be any delay, because ongoing metabolism in the blood will consume oxygen and may affect the results. Exposure to air (bubbles in the syringe) will also affect the results.

pH results are sometimes presented as hydrogen ion concentrations ($[H^+]$) and gas pressures can be expressed in either kPa or mmHg. This book uses pH and mmHg. To convert kPa to mmHg, multiply by 7.5. The conversion of pH to $[H^+]$ is more difficult since pH is a logarithmic scale. The conversion between these is shown in Tables 8.1(a) and 8.1(b).

Table 8.1(a)	The conversion of H^+ concentration to pH is given by the formula: $pH = -\log [H^+]$ where H^+ is measured in moles/litre	
	pH	**H^+ (nmol)**
Severe acidosis	7.00	100
Acidosis	7.30	50
Lower limit of normal	7.35	45
Normal	**7.40**	**40**
Upper limit of normal	7.45	36
Alkalosis	7.50	32
Severe alkalosis	7.80	16

Table 8.1(b)	The conversion gas pressure from kPa to mmHg is more straightforward—multiply by 7.5		
	kPa	**mmHg**	
	4.0	30	
	4.7	35	(lower limit of normal Pa_{CO_2})
Normal Pa_{CO_2}	**5.3**	**40**	
	6.0	45	(upper limit of normal Pa_{CO_2})
	8.0	60	
	10.0	75	
	10.7	80	(lower limit of normal Pa_{O_2})
Normal Pa_{O_2}	**12.0**	**90**	
	13.3	100	(upper limit of normal Pa_{O_2})

Carbon dioxide (Paco$_2$)

Carbon dioxide dissolves readily in water and rapidly diffuses from the blood into alveoli. In effect there is no difference in the partial pressures of carbon dioxide in the alveoli and pulmonary circulation, and the rate-limiting step for the removal of CO$_2$ from the body is alveolar ventilation. Arterial carbon dioxide tension (Paco$_2$) is therefore inversely proportional to alveolar ventilation (if ventilation doubles, the Paco$_2$ falls by 50% and vice versa). Not all of the tidal ventilation participates in alveolar gas exchange. Some is used up in the conducting airways (*anatomic dead space*) and some may go to underperfused alveoli (*alveolar dead space*). The sum of this 'wasted' ventilation is known as the *physiological dead space*. The proportion of the tidal volume that goes to functioning alveoli is sometimes called the 'effective alveolar ventilation'. While alveolar disease may increase the dead space, this is usually offset by an increase in total ventilation and does not alter the Paco$_2$. This can have profound effects on the load on the respiratory muscles, which have to maintain adequate effective alveolar ventilation by increasing either the tidal volume or respiratory frequency.

In hyperventilation the Paco$_2$ falls as carbon dioxide is 'blown off' or washed out of alveoli. This can be caused by anxiety (such as fear of the needle used to obtain the arterial blood sample) or by hypoxia that is stimulating ventilation. Hyperventilation is also a physiological response to metabolic acidosis (see below).

In the early stages of an asthma attack there may be a fall in Paco$_2$. This is because the initial physiological defect in acute asthma is thought to be a ventilation/perfusion mismatch and an increase in the work of breathing, causing a paradoxical increase in ventilation. In the later stages, as airflow obstruction increases, effective alveolar ventilation is reduced and the Paco$_2$ rises.

Hypoventilation is associated with a rise in Paco$_2$. This has several causes:

- severe airflow obstruction—overloading the respiratory 'pump'
- severe restrictive lung disease—also overloading the respiratory pump
- failure of the respiratory pump due to kyphoscoliosis or neuromuscular disease
- failure of central respiratory drive

Chronic obstructive pulmonary disease and acute severe asthma are common causes of hypercapnoea due to airflow obstruction. Obstructive sleep apnoea may cause intermittent hypoxia and hypercapnoea due to upper airways obstruction during sleep. Occasionally, morbid obesity will cause such an increase in respiratory work that hypoventilation occurs—particularly during sleep—and this may be difficult to distinguish from obstructive sleep apnoea. Ventilatory failure due to chest wall deformity or respiratory muscle disease is usually a late sign and suggests a poor prognosis.

Central hypoventilation is poorly understood but is sometimes associated with neurological disease. It also occurs in severe heart failure, causing Cheyne-Stokes respiration. Patients with severe chronic obstructive pulmonary disease sometimes become accustomed to chronically high $PaCO_2$ levels and have a reduced respiratory drive (the 'blue bloater' syndrome). It is important to recognise these patients because they depend on hypoxia to stimulate respiration and high doses of supplemental oxygen can cause a profound depression in their respiratory drive.

pH and bicarbonate

Dissolved carbon dioxide combines with water to produce bicarbonate and hydrogen ions according to the following equilibrium:

$$CO_2 + H_2O \rightleftharpoons H^+ + HCO_3^-$$

In other words, carbon dioxide acts as an acid (for more detailed explanation see *The Henderson-Hasselbalch equation*). An increase in $PaCO_2$ due to hypoventilation will drive the equilibrium to the right and cause an increase in H^+ ions (a fall in pH). This is a *respiratory acidosis*. Conversely, an increase in ventilation will lower $PaCO_2$ and cause a *respiratory alkalosis*.

Disturbances of acid–base balance from non-respiratory causes are known as *metabolic* disturbances. The change in pH is associated with the opposite change in $PaCO_2$ to that expected from a respiratory cause. A *metabolic acidosis* (for example, diabetic ketoacidosis) will be associated with a low $PaCO_2$ as ventilation is increased to 'blow-off' carbon dioxide in an attempt to raise the pH. A metabolic alkalosis (for example, prolonged vomiting) is associated with a raised $PaCO_2$ because the raised pH reduces ventilatory drive. The

THE HENDERSON-HASSELBALCH EQUATION

The Henderson-Hasselbalch equation appears to be beloved by biochemists and physiologists. Perhaps this is because it provides the opportunity to ask questions which students will invariably get wrong. To understand arterial blood gas and acid–base balance, all you really need to remember is that carbon dioxide dissolves in water to form a weak acid and bicarbonate ions. This constitutes a useful buffer system for the body since both sides of the equation are subject to homeostatic control. Carbon dioxide can be removed by increasing ventilation (rapid response) and bicarbonate can be adjusted by altering renal excretion (relatively slow response). Thus the body can manipulate this buffer system in health to respond to changes in acid–base balance.

Because the Henderson-Hasselbalch equation (sometimes known as the 'hassle' equation) is so popular with examiners it is presented here in a little more detail:

$$pH = 6.1 + \log \frac{HCO_3^-}{0.03 \times PCO_2}$$

where   6.1 is the negative logarithm of the dissociation constant of carbon dioxide (pKa)

0.03 is the solubility coefficient for CO_2 to convert PCO_2 in mmHg to mmol/L

HCO_3^- is in mmol

If the H^+ is expressed in nmol rather than pH the equation is simpler:

$$H^+ = \frac{24 \times PCO_2}{HCO_3^-}$$

Note that the hydrogen ion concentration is directly related to the ratio of carbon dioxide pressure and bicarbonate concentration. Normally the concentration of bicarbonate is 20 times that of carbon dioxide (normal $[HCO_3^-] = 24$ mmol, normal $[CO_2] = 0.03 \times 40 = 1.2$ mmol). In theory this is an inefficient buffer system—in an ideal buffer the ratio would be equal. However, the ability to adjust both PCO_2 and $[HCO_3^-]$ provides a powerful method of control.

expected changes in respiratory and metabolic disturbances can be worked out from Figure 8.1. We suggest that you draw this diagram whenever you are trying to work out a blood gas. More precise versions of this diagram exist (see *The Flenley acid–base diagram*) but they are harder to sketch on the back of an envelope.

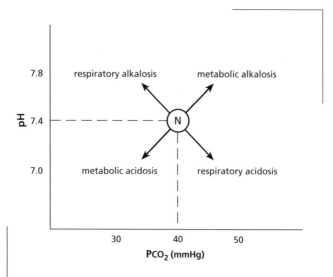

Figure 8.1 Patterns of change of P_{CO_2} and pH in respiratory and metabolic acid–base disorders. The circle 'N' indicates normality.

If a disturbance of acid–base balance persists, the body attempts to compensate for the disturbance. Respiratory compensation for metabolic disorders occurs by increasing or reducing ventilation as above—this is fairly rapid. Renal compensation for a primary respiratory disturbance occurs by the retention of bicarbonate ions, and takes a few days. It is important to remember that:

- the compensatory mechanisms attempt to restore a normal pH (7.40)
- the compensatory mechanisms rarely achieve full compensation and never overcompensate
- respiratory acidosis is compensated by a metabolic alkalosis (and vice versa)
- metabolic acidosis is compensated by a respiratory alkalosis (and vice versa)

THE FLENLEY ACID–BASE DIAGRAM

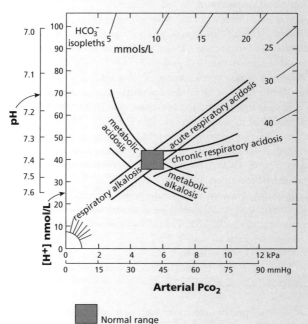

Normal range

Significance bands of single disturbances
in human whole blood in vivo

Figure 8.2 The Flenley acid–base diagram
From D. C. Flenley, 'Interpretation of blood gas and acid–base data', *British Journal of Hospital Medicine 1978*, 20(4), pp. 384–95. Used with permission of the publishers.

The scales on this diagram allow the acid–base status of a patient to be plotted with precision. The abnormality will be indicated by the zones. Note that the isopleths for HCO_3^- indicate that only one value of bicarbonate should be possible for each combination of Pco_2 and pH. This diagram can be very helpful in figuring out difficult acid–base problems.

Acute or chronic respiratory acidosis?

Most blood gas analysers do not measure the bicarbonate (HCO_3^-) concentration directly but calculate it from pH and $P\text{CO}_2$ using the Henderson-Hasselbalch equation. It follows that this is not strictly necessary for interpreting a blood gas because all the information is contained in the pH and $P\text{CO}_2$ values. However, the bicarbonate value is helpful since most people cannot calculate this from the Henderson-Hasselbalch equation by mental arithmetic. Pure respiratory changes in acid–base balance lead to small changes in HCO_3^-. Metabolic disturbances lead to much bigger changes in HCO_3^-. Thus an acute rise in $P\text{aCO}_2$ will cause a small rise in HCO_3^- because the equilibrium will be driven to the right. If the raised $P\text{aCO}_2$ persists, there will be a much bigger rise in HCO_3^- because of renal retention of bicarbonate (a compensatory metabolic alkalosis). This is extremely useful in distinguishing between acute and chronic ventilatory failure. The bicarbonate level is also useful for detecting mixed respiratory and metabolic acidosis/alkalosis. The following provide useful guides:

- Acute: for each 10 mmHg $P\text{CO}_2$ increase, pH decreases by 0.08, HCO_3^- increases by 1
- Chronic: for each 10 mmHg $P\text{CO}_2$ increase, pH decreases by 0.04, HCO_3^- increases by 3

Combined primary metabolic and respiratory disorders occasionally occur. These are characterised by a severe disturbance of pH, and abnormalities in both $P\text{CO}_2$ and HCO_3^-. The changes in $P\text{CO}_2$ and HCO_3^- tend to be in opposite directions and are also the opposite to those predicted by compensatory mechanisms:

- Combined metabolic/respiratory acidosis—low pH, high $P\text{CO}_2$, low HCO_3^-
- Combined metabolic/respiratory alkalosis—high pH, low $P\text{CO}_2$, high HCO_3^-

Theoretical concepts such as the 'standard' bicarbonate and the 'base excess' are also often provided from calculations on blood gas reports. These are intended to help the interpretation of acid–base disorders but in general they are more likely to confuse than help, and are best ignored. Note also that oxygen levels, although very important in arterial blood gas analysis, play no part in the interpretation of the acid–base status.

Oxygenation (Pa_{O_2})

Interpretation of the arterial oxygen tension (Pa_{O_2}) is more complicated than that of Pa_{CO_2}. Oxygen is much less soluble in water than
carbon dioxide and this means that:

- Oxygen diffuses poorly across alveolar membranes and there is
  a small pressure difference between the alveolar oxygen
  tension (PA_{O_2}) and that in arterial blood (Pa_{O_2}).
- A large alveolar area is required for oxygen transfer.
- Little oxygen is dissolved in body tissues. In the blood the vast
  majority of oxygen is carried bound to haemoglobin.

Despite the limitations to oxygen transfer, the haemoglobin circu-
lating through normal alveoli becomes nearly 100% saturated with
oxygen when a person breathes air at sea level. Increasing the oxygen
tension will therefore make little difference to the oxygen content of
the blood. The relationship between Pa_{O_2} and oxygen saturation is
described by the haemoglobin–oxygen dissociation curve (Fig. 8.3). It
will be seen that under normal conditions the Pa_{O_2} is on a plateau
which means that modest changes in oxygen tension make little
difference to haemoglobin saturation.

The Pa_{O_2} is sensitive to changes in both ventilation and alveolar
disease and thus almost any disease can cause hypoxia if sufficiently
severe. Reduced ventilation leads to a decrease in alveolar oxygen
tension (PA_{O_2}) and therefore a reduction in the Pa_{O_2}. The reduction
in ventilation is obvious from the rise in arterial carbon dioxide
tension (Pa_{CO_2}).

A low Pa_{O_2} in the presence of a normal Pa_{CO_2} indicates a problem
with gas transfer at the alveolar level or a shunt. This may be due to a

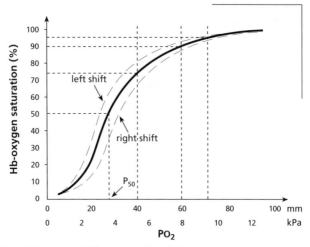

Figure 8.3 Haemoglobin–oxygen dissociation curve
The solid line describes the relationship between the partial pressures of
oxygen (Po_2) and haemoglobin–oxygen saturation for normal haemoglobin at
pH 7.4 and 37°C. A 'right shift' is caused by increased temperature, increased
carbon dioxide, acidosis and increased 2,3 diphosphoglycerate
concentrations—conditions found in exercising muscles where the shift to the
right allows more oxygen to be released to the tissues. A 'left shift' is caused
by the reverse conditions and increases oxygen binding to haemoglobin for a
given level of Po_2.

At normal levels of Pao_2 (70–100 mmHg, 9.3–13.3 kPa), haemoglobin is
more than 95% saturated. At 60 mmHg (8 kPa) haemoglobin is approximately
90% saturated. Below this the saturation falls steeply. At the normal venous
oxygen tension of 40 mmHg (5.3 kPa) saturation is 75%. The P_{50} is the oxygen
tension at which the haemoglobin is 50% saturated. This can be used to
describe the curve (a left or right shift) and for normal haemoglobin is
approximately 27 mmHg (3.6 kPa).

loss of alveolar area for gas exchange or thickening of the alveolar wall,
both of which increase the barrier to oxygen diffusion. More often it
is due to a ventilation/perfusion ($\dot{V}/\dot{Q}$) mismatch, whereby part of the
pulmonary circulation passes through the lungs without coming into
contact with oxygenated alveoli. Because of the oxygen-binding
characteristics of haemoglobin a small volume of deoxygenated blood

mixing with fully oxygenated blood (a 'shunt') leads to a disproportionate fall in the PaO_2. Although there may be a compensatory increase in ventilation in response to severe hypoxia, this is usually unable to restore the oxygen content of the blood to normal because the haemoglobin leaving the functioning alveolar capillaries is already nearly 100% saturated and cannot take much more oxygen. Similarly, increasing the inspired oxygen concentration will have little effect on the oxygen content if a shunt is present.

Common causes of a fall in PaO_2 with a normal (or low) $PaCO_2$ include:

- emphysema (which may also be associated with ventilatory failure)
- interstitial lung disease (for example, cryptogenic fibrosing alveolitis)
- severe pneumonia (an intrapulmonary shunt of blood through unventilated lung tissue)
- pulmonary embolism
- right-to-left cardiac shunt (cyanotic heart disease)

Alveolar-arterial oxygen (A-a) gradient

It is easy to interpret the PaO_2 if the $PaCO_2$ (and therefore ventilation) is normal and the patient is breathing normal (room) air. It is more difficult if the $PaCO_2$ is abnormal—is the abnormality in PaO_2 due to hypoventilation alone, or is there another pathological process? This issue can be resolved by estimating the oxygen tension difference between the alveoli and arterial blood (A-a gradient). You do not need to know many equations to interpret respiratory physiology but this one is worth learning:

$$\text{A-a gradient} = 150 - (PaO_2 + 1.25 \times PaCO_2) \text{ in mmHg}$$
$$\text{or} = 20 - (PaO_2 + 1.25 \times PaCO_2) \text{ in kPa}$$

The principle behind the A-a gradient calculation is that the alveolar oxygen tension (PAO_2) is equivalent to the inspired oxygen tension minus the oxygen that has been taken up by the blood. In the steady state the oxygen consumed is directly related to the carbon dioxide produced. The exact relationship between oxygen consumption and carbon dioxide production depends on the food being metabolised, but a reasonable approximation is 1.25 O_2 molecules for each CO_2 molecule. We know that the alveolar and arterial carbon dioxide tensions are the same because carbon dioxide diffuses so easily through the tissues ($PACO_2 = PaCO_2$). Therefore the oxygen taken up from the alveolus is $1.25 \times PaCO_2$.

Thus PAO_2 = inspired $PO_2 - (1.25 \times PaCO_2)$

Humidified air at sea-level contains approximately 150 mmHg (20 kPa) oxygen; therefore:

$$PAO_2 = 150 - (1.25 \times PaCO_2) \text{ mmHg}$$
$$\text{or} \quad PAO_2 = 20 - (1.25 \times PaCO_2) \text{ kPa}$$

In normal lungs the difference between the calculated PAO_2 and measured PaO_2 (the 'A-a gradient') is less than 15 mmHg (2 kPa). Values higher than this indicate alveolar disease or $\dot{V}/\dot{Q}$ mismatch. The A-a gradient should be normal in pure ventilatory disorders.

The A-a gradient can also be used to estimate the normal PaO_2 in a patient breathing supplemental oxygen or breathing at a different barometric pressure (altitude). The partial pressure of oxygen in inspired air is calculated from the following:

$$\text{Partial pressure of } O_2 = \text{barometric pressure} - (\text{water vapour pressure}) \times FiO_2$$

where FiO_2 = fraction of inspired oxygen, and water vapour pressure at body temperature = 47 mmHg (or 6.25 kPa).

The FiO_2 is known accurately only if the patient is breathing air or is intubated. However, some oxygen masks (for example, the Venturi type) allow a reasonably reliable estimate if they are set at the correct oxygen flow rate.

Respiratory failure

Type I respiratory failure is an isolated disorder of oxygenation (the $PaCO_2$ is normal) and is arbitrarily defined as a $PaO_2 < 60$ mmHg (8 kPa). Why 60 mmHg? Below this point on the haemoglobin–oxygen saturation curve the oxygen saturation begins to fall steeply and the oxygen content of blood rapidly decreases—see Figure 8.3.

Type II (or *hypercapnic*) respiratory failure is arbitrarily defined as $PaCO_2 > 50$ mmHg (6.7 kPa). Invariably this will be accompanied by a reduced PaO_2 (unless this has been corrected with supplemental oxygen).

The nomenclature 'type I' and 'type II' respiratory failure is often confusing and it is better to think of *hypoxic* and *ventilatory* (or hypercapnic) failure. Unfortunately the terms type I and II are widely used. To remember which is which: type I = one abnormal gas (PaO_2); type II = two abnormal gases (PaO_2 and $PaCO_2$).

Oxygen saturation

It should be obvious from the discussion above that PaO_2 does not directly measure blood oxygen *content*—just the arterial oxygen *tension*. The oxygen content is dependent on the haemoglobin concentration of the blood and the percentage haemoglobin-oxygen saturation. The oxygen saturation is often provided on arterial blood gas reports. Often this is not measured but estimated from the PO_2 and pH, assuming normal haemoglobin–oxygen binding characteristics. This assumption is not always correct—see below.

Oxygen saturation can be measured non-invasively using a pulse oximeter. Pulse oximeters estimate the percentage of oxygenated haemoglobin in arterial blood from the absorption of light in the red and infra-red spectra, using a probe on a finger or ear lobe. This is extremely useful for monitoring the oxygenation of patients without the need for repeated arterial puncture. Pulse oximeters are reasonably accurate (to within ± 3%) at high saturations, but are less accurate below about 80% saturation. There are several pitfalls with oximetry and it is important to be aware of these.

The relationship between PaO_2 and saturation is described by the haemoglobin–oxygen dissociation curve (Fig. 8.3). This shows that oxygen saturation is relatively insensitive to changes in oxygen tension around the normal PaO_2. Thus pulse oximetry may be normal despite significant problems with gas transfer. Below about 60 mmHg the slope becomes steep and a small change in PaO_2 may cause a large change in saturation (and therefore oxygen content).

The oxygen saturation also gives no indication of the adequacy of ventilation. Patients can be retaining carbon dioxide despite normal or near-normal oxygen saturations. This is particularly true in patients with chronic obstructive pulmonary disease who are given supplemental oxygen during an acute exacerbation. The extra oxygen may maintain or improve their oxygen saturations but reduce the hypoxic drive to ventilation. Ventilation falls and the resulting carbon dioxide retention and respiratory acidosis may be fatal.

Oximeters can be fooled by abnormal haemoglobin. Carboxyhaemoglobin (COHb) has similar light-absorption characteristics to oxyhaemoglobin. Patients with carbon monoxide poisoning have high oxygen saturation readings despite severe hypoxaemia (as indeed they do not appear to be cyanosed on clinical examination). Methaemoglobin (MetHb) also interferes with the spectral characteristics of the blood and tends to lead to saturation readings of around 85%.

COHb and MetHb also lead to errors in haemoglobin–oxygen saturation estimations from the P_{O_2}. Since the P_{O_2} reflects only the oxygen tension and not the oxygen content of the blood, it may be normal despite the presence of either COHb or MetHb. Calculations which assume that the haemoglobin is normal will therefore overestimate oxygen saturation. The true oxygen saturation can be measured accurately with a co-oximeter, which also measures the COHb and MetHb levels. Some machines now combine a co-oximeter with blood gas analysis and avoid this problem.

CHAPTER SUMMARY

→ The Pa_{CO_2} is a measure of ventilation. A doubling of the Pa_{CO_2} indicates a halving of ventilation and vice versa.

→ The Pa_{O_2} reflects both ventilation and pulmonary gas exchange. If both the Pa_{O_2} and Pa_{CO_2} are abnormal the A-a gradient is useful in finding out whether there is a problem with gas exchange in addition to ventilation.

→ In a *respiratory acidosis*, the fall in pH is due to CO_2 retention because of hypoventilation. Metabolic compensation occurs by the renal retention of HCO_3^-.

→ In a *metabolic acidosis*, respiratory compensation occurs rapidly by increased ventilation and reduction in the Pa_{CO_2}.

→ Pulse oximetry can be useful to monitor oxygenation, but is insensitive to problems with pulmonary gas exchange and does not help assess the adequacy of ventilation or the development of a respiratory acidosis.

Clinical examples

Patient 8A: age 72, male

History: COPD—acute exacerbation. This arterial blood gas measurement was obtained while the patient was breathing 2 litres of oxygen/minute by facial mask.

	Normal range	Measured
pH	7.37–7.42	(7.44)
P_{CO_2} mmHg	35–45	(54)
P_{O_2} mmHg	70–100	(60)
HCO_3^- mmol/L	23–28	(36)

Interpretation: The patient has a known history of COPD and presents with a deterioration in symptoms. The arterial blood gas measurement has been obtained shortly after admission to hospital while the patient is being treated with additional oxygen (F_{IO_2} = 2 litres by mask). There is no acidosis despite the elevated P_{CO_2}. In fact the pH is slightly raised. This suggests that he has a compensated respiratory acidosis; that is, he has a long standing type II respiratory failure. The pH may have risen above 7.4 either because of the anxiety associated with the admission and arterial puncture, or because the treatment he has already received is helping him to ventilate more than before. (The alternative explanation—that he has a primary metabolic alkalosis which is compensated by hypoventilation—is extremely unlikely in view of the clinical history and the degree of hypoxia.) He remains hypoxaemic despite the additional oxygen. The bicarbonate measurement is high, consistent with a compensatory response to chronic ventilatory failure.

Patient 8B: age 30, male

History: Acute presentation with dyspnoea.
    Arterial blood gas was taken while the patient was breathing air.

	Normal range	Measured
pH	7.37–7.42	(7.33)
P_{CO_2} mmHg	35–45	(24)
P_{O_2} mmHg	70–100	(111)
HCO_3^- mmol/L	23–28	(12)

Interpretation: The patient is acidotic but has a low P_{CO_2}. This indicates a metabolic acidosis with respiratory compensation. The hyperventilation has raised the P_{O_2} above normal. The A-a gradient is normal ($150 - (111 + 1.25 \times 24) = 9$), indicating that there is unlikely to be a problem with gas exchange. This patient was in diabetic ketoacidosis. The acidosis of this condition causes compensatory hyperventilation and a sensation of dyspnoea ('air hunger'). Air hunger can be mistaken for acute respiratory distress unless a blood gas is done.

Patient 8C: age 70, male

History: Acute presentation to the emergency department with haemoptysis and dyspnoea.

   Arterial blood gas was taken while the patient was breathing air.

	Normal range	Measured
pH	7.37–7.42	(7.50)
P_{CO_2} mmHg	35–45	(31)
P_{O_2} mmHg	70–100	88
HCO_3^- mmol/L	23–28	24

Interpretation: The pH is raised and the P_{CO_2} is reduced, indicating a respiratory alkalosis. This has not yet been compensated by renal bicarbonate excretion (the HCO_3^- remains in the low–normal range). The P_{O_2} is normal, but the A-a gradient is raised ($150 - (81 + 1.25 \times 31) = 30$), indicating a significant abnormality with gas exchange. Hypoxaemia does not normally cause an increased respiratory drive until the P_{O_2} is around 60 mmHg. The cause of the respiratory alkalosis (increased ventilation) could be anxiety, or an altered perception of the work of breathing (due to altered lung compliance caused by the underlying disorder).

A chest X-ray showed extensive abnormal shadowing over the right lung field. It was not clear if this shadowing was caused by blood (associated with the haemoptysis), pneumonia or another underlying disease.

Patient 8D: age 18, female

History: Acute presentation to the emergency department with chest tightness and dyspnoea over 4 hours. On examination she is distressed, tired and speaking in short sentences. Respiratory rate 28/min. Widespread wheeze.

This arterial blood gas was taken while the patient was breathing 6 L/min oxygen via face mask.

	Normal range	Measured
pH	7.37–7.42	(7.31)
P_{CO_2} mmHg	35–45	(49)
P_{O_2} mmHg	70–100	(115)
HCO_3^- mmol/L	23–28	26

Interpretation: The pH is low and the P_{CO_2} is raised, indicating a respiratory acidosis. The normal bicarbonate level as well as the clinical setting (acute asthma) indicate that this is acute. Despite her high ventilatory rate she is unable to blow off CO_2. Her P_{O_2} is difficult to interpret because she is breathing supplemental oxygen, and it is impossible to calculate the inspired concentration. However, the P_{O_2} is suspiciously low for someone on high-flow oxygen; this suggests that she is having difficulty with oxygenation. This is a medical emergency and she needs to be treated aggressively—preferably in an intensive care unit.

Patient 8E: age 37, female

History: Lifelong mild asthma. Last admission to hospital as a child. Presents to the emergency department with history of 3 weeks of troublesome wheeze with increasing dyspnoea and chest tightness for 24 hours. She became worried and called an ambulance. On examination she is anxious and distressed. Speaking in short sentences. Respiratory rate 18/min. Peak expiratory flow 150 L/min (previous best unknown).

An arterial blood gas was taken immediately on arrival while the patient was breathing room air.

	Normal range	Measured
pH	7.37–7.42	7.37
P_{CO_2} mmHg	35–45	43
P_{O_2} mmHg	70–100	91
HCO_3^- mmol/L	23–28	27

Interpretation: At first sight the arterial blood gas results appear to be normal and seem to confirm the impression that this lady has mild asthma and anxiety. The warning sign is the P_{CO_2} which, though in the normal range, is higher than would be expected for an anxious young patient. The A-a gradient is low (5 mmHg) which would also be unusual for a patient with mild asthma. Further enquiry revealed that she had been given oxygen to breathe in the ambulance and that this had been stopped only 2–3 minutes before the blood gas measurement. In fact, the high–normal P_{CO_2} indicates that she is developing ventilatory failure; she may also develop severe hypoxia now that she is breathing room air.

Patient 8F: age 19, male

History: This patient with Duchenne muscular dystrophy and who has been wheelchair-bound for 7 years presents with respiratory distress at midnight. He has no history of respiratory problems but has recurrent urinary tract infections and had commenced antibiotics for this the morning before his admission.

An arterial blood gas was taken shortly after arrival while he was breathing room air.

	Normal range	Measured
pH	7.35–7.45	(7.21)
P_{CO_2} mmHg	35–45	(81)
P_{O_2} mmHg	70–100	(44)
HCO_3^- mmol/L	23–28	(36)

Interpretation: He has a respiratory acidosis (raised P_{CO_2} and low pH). He is not as acidotic as would be expected for such a high P_{CO_2} and the HCO_3^- is high, indicating that he has acute or chronic respiratory failure. His A-a gradient is not increased, indicating that this is purely a ventilatory problem.

His chest X-ray showed small lung volumes but no evidence of pneumonia. The cause of his acute deterioration was thought to be the increased metabolic demand caused by the urinary tract infection, resulting in increased oxygen consumption and carbon dioxide production, which had overloaded his respiratory system. He was treated successfully with non-invasive ventilation acutely and continuing nocturnal support ventilation long-term. When well his FEV_1 was only 0.4 litres (19% predicted) and it is surprising that he had not developed respiratory symptoms before this—this is often the case in these very disabled patients who are unable to stress their respiratory system with exercise.

Patient 8G: age 57, male

History: Previously healthy smoker. One-week history of upper respiratory tract infection followed by a 36-hour history of cough, fever and dyspnoea. In respiratory distress with a respiratory rate 36/minute. Clinical evidence of a right basal pneumonia was confirmed on chest X-ray.

Initial arterial blood gas while breathing 2 L/min supplemental oxygen via face mask. Repeat measurements taken while on 10 L/min using a rebreathing mask.

	Normal range	Measured (1)	Measured (2)
Inspired oxygen (L/min)		2	10
pH	7.35–7.45	(7.33)	(7.34)
P_{CO_2} mmHg	35–45	(27)	(32)
P_{O_2} mmHg	70–100	(51)	(58)
HCO_3^- mmol/L	23–28	(22)	24

Interpretation: He has a severe type I (hypoxic) respiratory failure. He is slightly acidotic but his P_{CO_2} is low, excluding a respiratory acidosis. His HCO_3^- is slightly low, consistent with an early metabolic acidosis. The cause of this is most likely tissue hypoxia due to his hypoxaemia and poor perfusion of peripheral tissues. Despite the high flow oxygen, there is little increase in PaO_2, suggesting that the problem with gas exchange is due to the shunting of blood through the consolidated pneumonic lung. This blood does not come into contact with ventilated alveoli and will remain hypoxaemic regardless of the concentration of inspired oxygen. The blood flowing through the normal lung is already nearly 100% saturated with oxygen and cannot take up more oxygen to compensate for the deoxygenated blood coming from the pneumonic lung.

Chapter 9

Cardiopulmonary exercise tests

Why assess a patient's exercise capability and responses to exercise?

Spirometry and most other lung function tests assess lung function using maximum expiratory/inspiratory manoeuvres at rest, but, although providing very useful information, the procedures are unnatural. More often than not, patients complain of dyspnoea during exercise. A number of tests to assess the patient's performance while exercising have been developed. There are three main reasons for performing an exercise test:

1. to identify a cardiac or respiratory cause for exercise limitation
2. to quantify functional disability
3. to assess the response to treatment

Numerous patterns of exercise and variables monitored have been used over the years. Currently there are two types of test used to assess exercise, each with very definite roles. All exercise tests can be limited by other medical problems such as joint pain, intermittent claudication or angina.

Simple measures of exercise capacity

The most widely used of these tests are the 6-minute walking test and the shuttle test. In both tests patients are asked to exercise in a set pattern and the primary measurements made are:

- the distance walked
- the extent of any fall in oxygenation, as measured by a pulse oximeter
- symptoms of dyspnoea before and after exercise using an index such as the Borg scale (Table 9.1)

Table 9.1	The original Borg scale has been modified to make this 12-point scale to grade the severity of dyspnoea on exertion.
0	Nothing at all
0.5	Very very slight (just noticeable)
1	Very slight
2	Slight
3	Moderate
4	Somewhat severe
5	Severe
6	
7	Very severe
8	
9	Very very severe (almost maximal)
10	Maximal

Six-minute walk test

This is the simplest of the tests and requires no equipment other than a timer and ideally a portable pulse oximeter. The subject walks as far as they can at their own pace for 6 minutes on a set course (such as a hospital corridor). They are free to stop and rest at any time. Heart rate and oxygen saturation are measured just before and at the end of exercise.

This test is reproducible and is effective for monitoring the functional change in an individual in response to disease progression or response to treatment. It may also point to the underlying disorder. A fall in oxygen saturation of more than 5% is a strong indicator of a respiratory problem. Conversely an excessive heart rate response with no fall in oxygen saturation suggests that the patient is either very unfit or has a cardiac problem. (For further information see 'ATS statement: guidelines for the six-minute walk test', *American Journal of Respiratory and Critical Care Medicine*, 2002, 166, pp. 111–17.)

Shuttle test

In this test the individual is asked to walk back and forth around two points which are set 9 m apart (to allow 0.5 m to turn around—hence 10 m for each shuttle). The speed at which they walk is controlled by an audiocassette tape and is increased progressively. Patients continue shuttling until they cannot keep up with the tape or until they have to stop to recover their breath (or for other reasons such as weakness of the legs).

This test is a standardised and externally paced walking test and has good reproducibility, though it needs an experienced supervisor to ensure that it is performed adequately. A 12-level protocol covers a wide range of walking speeds to accommodate patients with minimal disability as well as those more severely disabled. (Further details of the methodology of the shuttle test can be found in S. J. Singh, M. D. L. Morgan, S. Scott, D. Walters & A. E. Hardman, 'Development of a shuttle walking test of disability in patients with chronic airways disease', *Thorax* 1992, 47, pp. 1019–24.)

Progressive exercise testing

In this type of exercise test the subject is asked to carry out progressively increasing workloads of exercise while their respiration is monitored breath by breath; their cardiovascular responses are also observed by recording their heart rate and ECG continuously during the exercise period and into recovery. These tests can be carried out to a varying degree of sophistication, and can include metabolic measurements, repeated arterial blood gas analysis via an arterial line and continuous blood pressure measurement using the arterial line or non-invasive systems (most laboratories do not use arterial lines).

The test can be carried out on either a cycle ergometer or a treadmill. The cycle ergometer allows an accurate assessment of workload but is an unfamiliar form of exercise for many patients. The treadmill provides more natural exercise, but it is difficult to assess workload because this will depend on the patient's weight and walking efficiency. The subject may exercise to achieve a preset target oxygen uptake ($\dot{V}O_2$) or keep going until they are unable to continue, to a maximal oxygen uptake ($\dot{V}O_2max$). Subjects may stop exercising because of dyspnoea, tiredness of the legs or other symptoms. Occasionally the test will be stopped by the supervising health professional because the predicted maximal heart rate is achieved, or because dangerous signs such as cardiac arrythmias or a fall in blood pressure have occurred.

Such exercise is a test of the three components involved in heavy physical exercise:

1. respiration
2. the cardiovascular system (both the heart and peripheral circulation)
3. the condition of the peripheral musculature

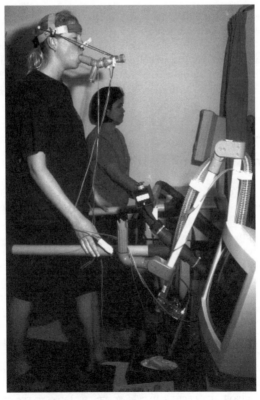

Figure 9.1 A subject on a treadmill instrumented to undergo a progressive cardiopulmonary exercise test

Modern exercise systems can produce a wealth of data and it is easy to lose sight of the purpose of the test. In most laboratories progressive exercise tests are used with one of the following aims:

- to distinguish between cardiac and respiratory causes for exercise limitation. In this situation the test is a pointer and cannot give an unequivocal answer. Exercise tests can also be used in patients complaining of exertional dyspnoea and who have no evidence of either cardiac or respiratory disease on screening. In this situation the test may suggest deconditioning, psychogenic breathlessness or underlying disease, classically pulmonary hypertension (rare).
- to quantify functional disability and to assess the patient's maximal level of fitness—the maximal oxygen uptake, usually measured as maximal oxygen uptake per kilogram body weight per minute (mL O_2/kg/min). Common uses are in the assessment of patients for pulmonary resection and for cardiac transplant.
- to assess the response to treatment. This is an expensive test and most units will prefer to use one of the simpler tests such as a shuttle test or a six-minute walk.

It is important to note that the results of exercise testing may indicate the organ system limiting exercise capacity, but will not provide a diagnosis. In many patients there may be a combination of factors (such as skeletal muscle deconditioning in patients with advanced cardiac disease).

Risks of exercise testing

The risks of exercise tests are low in most patients. However, exercise tests should not be performed in patients with acute myocardial infarction, unstable angina, uncontrolled symptomatic arrythmias, uncontrolled heart failure, severe aortic stenosis or acute pulmonary embolism/deep venous thrombosis. It is relatively contraindicated in patients with significant pulmonary hypertension, severe arterial hypertension, severe left main-stem coronary artery disease and hypertrophic cardiomyopathy.

Measurements

Most systems measure respiratory frequency, tidal volume, oxygen consumption and carbon dioxide production. Although each variable is calculated for each breath there is considerable breath-to-breath variability and most systems provide a running average over a set number of breaths (some collect the exhaled air in a mixing chamber or Douglas bag). Heart rate and oxygen saturation are monitored continuously. From these the following can be calculated:

- *Oxygen uptake ($\dot{V}O_2$)*: the oxygen consumption expressed as litres of oxygen per minute. It is derived by multiplying the measured oxygen consumption (a running average) by the respiratory frequency.
  - $\dot{V}O_2$ *peak*: the oxygen uptake at the peak of exercise. In a truly maximal exercise test this is the same as $\dot{V}O_2$ max, the maximum achievable oxygen uptake.
  - $\dot{V}O_2$/*kg body weight*: the oxygen consumption divided by body weight—this is an attempt to normalise for weight.
- *CO_2 production ($\dot{V}CO_2$)*: the volume of CO_2 produced each minute, derived from measuring exhaled CO_2 breath by breath and multiplying by the respiratory frequency.
- *Respiratory exchange ratio (RER)*: the ratio of carbon dioxide production to oxygen consumption, $\dot{V}CO_2/\dot{V}O_2$. This is sometimes called the *respiratory quotient* (RQ) which is actually the ratio of carbon dioxide production to oxygen consumption in the metabolising tissues. The RER and the RQ are the same if the patient is at steady state but may differ in a changing situation (such as increasing exercise).
- *Minute ventilation ($\dot{V}E$)*: the product of the tidal volume and respiratory frequency. For any given workload or given level of oxygen consumption, minute ventilation can be predicted from normal values. Excessive ventilation for a given workload is seen in both respiratory and cardiac disease. As a rule grossly excessive ventilation for a given workload is suggestive of major respiratory disease.
- *Oxygen pulse ($\dot{V}O_2$ pulse)*: oxygen consumption divided by heart rate provides a measure of the oxygen delivery per heart cycle and thus an indirect measure of stroke volume (this involves several assumptions). During progressive exercise stroke volume increases markedly and failure of oxygen pulse to increase appropriately is highly suggestive of a limited cardiac reserve. This pattern is classically seen in severe pulmonary hypertension and left ventricular failure.
- *Tidal volume*: the volume of each breath. The pattern of tidal volume response to exercise can suggest the aetiology of the

dyspnoea. For example, in severe restrictive lung disease the respiratory rate is high and tidal volume does not increase significantly on exercise. This response is an attempt to limit the work of breathing which would increase dramatically (due to the 'stiff' lungs) if a large tidal volume breath was taken.

- *Pulse oximetry*: direct measurement of arterial PO_2 would be ideal. In practice most laboratories use pulse oximetry. Healthy subjects do not desaturate during exercise (elite athletes are an occasional exception to this rule). Even in respiratory disease desaturation on exercise is not inevitable—many patients stop exercising from dyspnoea or fatigue before this occurs. Desaturation indicates a major failure of either the respiratory system (the most common clinical situation) or the cardiovascular system to increase its ability to load and/or transport oxygen.

Interpretation

The responses of the various respiratory and cardiovascular variables are usually compared to workload. The workload can be calculated directly (this is easier with cycle ergometers), or the oxygen uptake can be used as a substitute measure. The other variables such as minute ventilation or heart rate can be related to workload or oxygen uptake and compared with a predicted range of normal values.

In health, exercise tolerance is limited by the ability of the cardiovascular system to supply oxygen to the musculature. When the ability to supply oxygen to the muscles is exceeded, any additional work is generated by anaerobic metabolism, producing lactic acid. In order to compensate for this metabolic acidosis, ventilation increases and carbon dioxide is eliminated at a greater rate than would be expected with respect to oxygen uptake. This point can often be seen on a graph of ventilation, or CO_2 elimination plotted against oxygen uptake (Fig. 9.2) and is called the *anaerobic threshold* (also known as the *lactate threshold*). Anaerobic exercise is difficult to maintain, and eventually the subject tires and stops exercising. In health, the anaerobic threshold usually occurs around 60–70% of the maximum oxygen uptake ($\dot{V}o_2max$).

Even at maximum exercise, there is significant respiratory reserve in healthy subjects. The theoretical *maximum voluntary ventilation* (MVV) can be measured by asking the subject to breathe as hard and

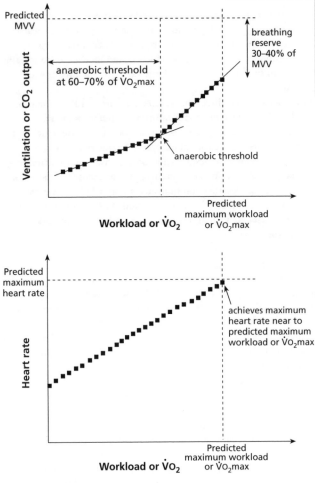

Figure 9.2 Normal exercise physiology
Two graphs are plotted, showing the normal increase in ventilation (or CO_2 output) with increasing workload (top diagram). The anaerobic threshold is indicated as a change in the slope—a greater increase in ventilation or CO_2 output relative to the increase in workload. Note that ventilation does not reach the predicted maximum, leaving a 'breathing reserve' of 30–40%. The bottom diagram shows a linear increase in heart rate with workload, which reaches the maximum predicted at the end of exercise.

fast as possible for 10–15 seconds and extrapolating the result to 1 minute, or estimated by multiplying the FEV_1 by 35. The peak ventilation achieved during maximal exercise is usually 30–40% less than the MVV. This is known as the *breathing reserve*. A reduced breathing reserve suggests there may be a ventilatory limit to exercise (see below). Arterial oxygen saturation (and Pao_2 if measured) should not fall, even at maximum exercise.

In general, if the patient achieves a maximum oxygen uptake ($\dot{V}o_2$max) and heart rate which are close to the predicted maximums the test result is probably normal. If either of these is not achieved it is important to consider the reasons: did the patient stop prematurely or have an abnormal physiological limit to exercise? It is important to record the patient's reason for stopping, as this may indicate a problem unrelated to the cardiopulmonary system (such as joint pain). The severity of dyspnoea can be estimated using a scale such as the Borg scale (Table 9.1). One complication in interpretation is that the range of 'normal' for exercise tolerance is poorly defined. Athletes may achieve an oxygen uptake in excess of 200% predicted.

In patients with a *cardiovascular limit* to exercise (see Fig. 9.3), the heart rate response is usually excessive. The predicted maximum heart rate is reached early on and the patient stops exercising before the predicted maximum oxygen uptake is reached. The heart is unable to increase the stroke-volume in response to exercise and the *oxygen pulse* (the oxygen uptake divided by the heart-rate), which is a substitute measure for stroke-volume, is low. Exercise may be accompanied by ECG abnormalities such as ischaemia or arrythmias. Occasionally, exercise may be limited by an inability to increase the heart rate (for example, conduction abnormalities or beta-blocking drugs). This is usually obvious. Providing there is no respiratory problem, ventilation is not excessive and the *breathing reserve* is increased. The anaerobic threshold (if this can be detected) may occur early— below 50% of the $\dot{V}o_2$max because of the inability of the circulation to supply oxygen to the exercising muscles (Fig. 9.3).

In unfit (*deconditioned*) patients, the cardiovascular system is less able to sustain a workload because the skeletal and cardiac muscles are out of condition. The features are therefore similar to a cardiovascular limitation. The oxygen pulse (an indirect measure of cardiac stroke volume) is an indicator of fitness—a trained subject can achieve higher workloads because the cardiac output and oxygen delivery for a given heart rate is higher. Unfit patients may have a reduced oxygen

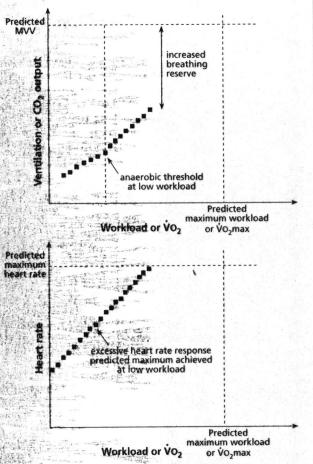

Figure 9.3 Cardiovascular limitation to exercise
The top graph indicates that the anaerobic threshold occurs early because the circulatory system is unable to supply sufficient oxygen to the tissues—hence anaerobic metabolism starts earlier than expected. The breathing reserve at peak exertion is increased—the respiratory system is not limiting exercise and is capable of much more ventilation. The bottom graph indicates a greater than expected heart-rate response to exercise (the slope is steeper) and this reaches a maximum early, confirming that it is the cardiovascular system which is limiting the exercise tolerance. This can be very difficult to distinguish from deconditioning (see Fig. 9.4).

pulse, but this should increase in a near-normal fashion with workload (it may not reach the predicted value because the patient stops too soon). A low *anaerobic threshold* may also indicate severe deconditioning (Fig. 9.4).

Distinguishing deconditioning from other causes of exercise limitation (particularly cardiovascular disease) is extremely difficult and may sometimes be impossible. Most severe cardiac and respiratory diseases result in deconditioning of the musculature and the results of an exercise test may reflect this as well as the underlying diagnosis. The distinction is not helped by the poor definition of 'normal'. An extremely low oxygen pulse (less than 50% predicted) at peak exercise is a clue to an underlying cardiovascular condition, but less severe abnormalities may simply be due to lack of fitness.

If there is a *respiratory* limit to exercise, a number of abnormalities may be seen. Most often, ventilation increases excessively with respect to workload or oxygen uptake. The patient may reach the predicted MVV and the breathing reserve will be low. The predicted maximum heart rate may not be achieved. The anaerobic threshold is not detected because the patient is unable to increase ventilation further in response to lactic acidosis (Fig. 9.5). A fall in oxygen saturation is not always seen, but is a strong pointer to a respiratory problem if it occurs. Rarely, oxygen saturation may increase during exercise because the increase in cardiac output improves ventilation-perfusion matching. If the exercise system is capable of calculating the dead space to tidal volume ratio (V_D/V_T), this ratio should fall in healthy subjects during exercise as tidal volume (V_T) increases, but in patients with respiratory disease V_D/V_T is likely to remain the same or even increase because more of the ventilation is 'wasted' (there is an increase in dead space (V_D)). Accurate assessment of V_D/V_T requires measurement of arterial Pa_{CO_2} during exercise. Some systems use the end-tidal CO_2 as a non-invasive approximation of Pa_{CO_2} but this assumption may not be true in patients with respiratory disease.

Table 9.2 summarises the common abnormalities in patients with deconditioning, cardiovascular and respiratory limitations to exercise. It is important to look at the responses throughout exercise as well as the maximum values achieved. They should be interpreted in the context of the clinical presentation. The reason for stopping exercise should also be borne in mind when interpreting the results—was this really a maximum exercise test?

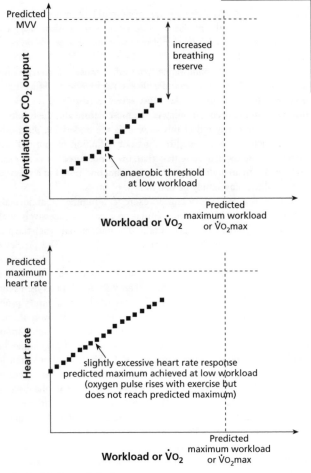

Figure 9.4 Deconditioning

These graphs are similar to those in Figure 9.3. The top diagram is almost identical, but the bottom graph shows a less steep heart-rate response. The predicted maximum heart rate is not achieved because the peripheral musculature limits exercise more than the cardiovascular system does. This distinction can be very difficult and often impossible to make in the clinical setting. To complicate matters, most patients with severe cardiovascular or respiratory disease will develop deconditioning of the peripheral musculature because of their inability to exercise.

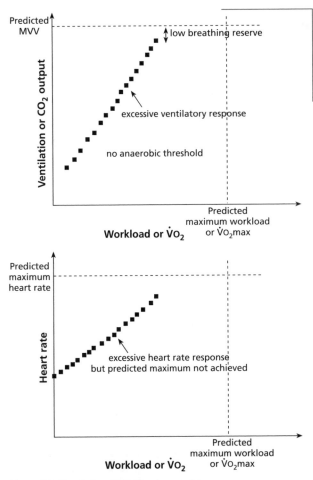

Figure 9.5 Respiratory limitation to exercise
Ventilation in response to exercise is excessive. Despite approaching
near-maximal ventilation the patient achieves only a low peak $\dot{V}O_2$. The
breathing reserve is low—it is the inability to increase ventilation which is
limiting exertion. There is no anaerobic threshold because the patient cannot
increase ventilation in response to lactic acidosis. The heart-rate response may
be excessive, but the predicted maximum is not achieved because the patient
stops exercising due to their respiratory limitation. Oxygen saturations are not
shown on these graphs, but a progressive fall in saturation with exercise would
be a strong pointer to a respiratory limitation.

Table 9.2	Basic patterns of exercise responses		
Variable	Deconditioned subject	Cardiovascular limitation	Respiratory limitation
$\dot{V}o_2$max	Low	Low	Low
Breathing reserve	High	High	Low
Heart rate	High	High	Low
$\dot{V}o_2$ pulse	Low/normal	Low	Normal/low

A WARNING!

Almost any variable can be plotted breath by breath against any other variable, leading to a plethora of graphical data and the risk of confusion or a temptation to find 'abnormalities' of questionable importance. It is essential to have a clear-cut question that you wish the exercise test to answer, such as assessing the patient's suitability for surgical resection, or determining which system is the main contributor to exercise limitation. Treat any unexpected 'abnormal' findings with deep suspicion.

CHAPTER SUMMARY

→ Exercise tests fall into two categories:
   – simple tests of exercise capacity such as the six-minute walk test or shuttle test
   – sophisticated, progressive exercise tests, usually to maximal effort, during which a wide variety of cardiac and pulmonary variables are measured continuously to assess the pattern of cardiorespiratory limitation on exercise.
→ When ordering an exercise test, it is essential to have a clearly formulated clinical question you wish the test to answer, and order the correct test for that clinical indication or question.
→ The results of progressive exercise tests are often not clearcut and so must always be interpreted within that individual patient's clinical situation by the individual ordering the test, not blindly interpreted by the laboratory staff.
→ If you are not sure whether an exercise test will help in a given clinical situation or if the result does not make sense, do not

hesitate to discuss the situation with a clinical respiratory physician/physiologist. The result is rarely black and white; we all find interpreting exercise tests challenging and, in all honesty, sometimes near impossible!

. . . see over for clinical examples

Clinical examples

Patient 9A: age 43, male, height 1.84 m, weight 102 kg

History: Sedentary man with history of sarcoidosis 15 years previously, from which he made an uneventful recovery. Complains of increasing dyspnoea climbing hills and stairs over several months. Normal chest X-ray. Family history of coronary artery disease.

		Predicted	Measured	% predicted
Spirometry	FEV_1 litres	3.99	3.78	95
	FVC litres	5.34	4.80	90
	FEV_1/FVC %	74	79	
	$FEF_{25-75\%}$ L/s	3.96	3.58	90
Lung volumes	TLC litres	7.39	6.95	94
(plethysmograph)	RV litres	2.22	2.13	96
	RV/TLC %	31	31	
	FRC litres	3.70	2.68	73
	VC litres	5.34	4.82	90
Gas transfer				
DLco mL/min/mmHg		31.4	36.2	115
DLco/VA mL/min/mmHg/L		4.30	5.68	132
VA litres		6.37		

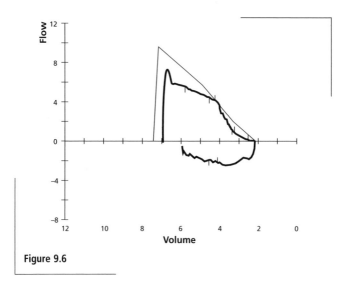

Figure 9.6

Interpretation: The lung function test results are normal. The flow-volume loop shows a 'knee', which is a normal variant most often seen in young women. A progressive exercise test was ordered to attempt to identify the cause of his dyspnoea.

Exercise report

Resting data: heart rate 77/min, $\dot{V}O_2$ 0.386 L/min, respiratory rate 15/min

The patient exercised on a treadmill for 10 minutes at a speed of 4 km/h. The slope was progressively increased by 2% each minute up to 18%. He did not desaturate. He had no dyspnoea at all at the end of the test.

On peak exertion

	Predicted	Measured	% predicted
Oxygen uptake			
$\dot{V}O_2$ mL/kg/min	36.3	(21.2)	(58)
$\dot{V}O_2$ L/min	2.82	(2.17)	(77)
Oxygen saturation		97%	

	Predicted	Measured	% predicted
Cardiovascular response			
Heart rate beats/min	172	133	(78)
O_2 pulse mL/beat	18.9	16.3	86
Ventilatory response			
Ventilation L/min	132.3*	50.6	38
Breathing reserve		62%	
Respiratory exchange ratio		0.95	

(*maximum ventilation predicted from $35 \times FEV_1$)

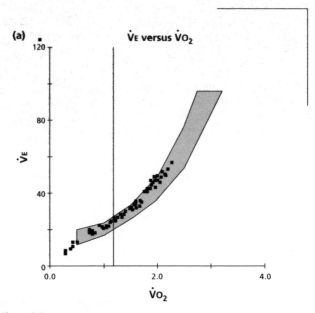

Figure 9.7

Four graphs are shown (many more could be plotted). (a) The rise in ventilation ($\dot{V}E$) with increasing oxygen uptake ($\dot{V}O_2$)—an indirect measure of workload. The response is within the normal (shaded) area.

(continued)

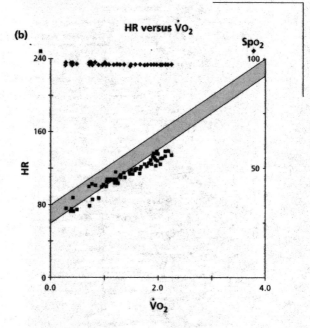

Figure 9.7 (continued)
(b) The heart rate response (HR) to oxygen uptake ($\dot{V}o_2$). The response is at the lower normal range. This graph also plots the change in oxygen saturation at the top of the graph—the scale for this is on the right. There is no significant desaturation.

(continued)

McGraw-Hill's pocket guide to lung function tests

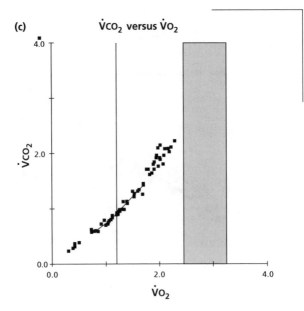

Figure 9.7 (continued)
(c) The carbon dioxide output ($\dot{V}CO_2$) versus oxygen uptake ($\dot{V}O_2$). Since the carbon dioxide output is proportional to the ventilation, the graph looks very similar to (a) and does not add much more information. The vertical line on this graph indicates where the computer detects a change in the slope of the plot. This indicates the anaerobic threshold (increased carbon dioxide produced anaerobic metabolism in the exercising muscles). The same line is shown in (a). The position of the anaerobic threshold in this case is not very convincing. The shaded area on the right indicates the predicted maximum $\dot{V}O_2$ which the patient does not achieve.

(continued)

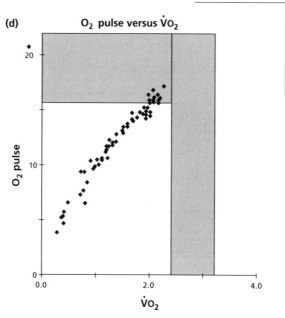

(d) O_2 **pulse versus** $\dot{V}O_2$

Figure 9.7 (continued)
(d) Oxygen pulse versus oxygen uptake. The oxygen pulse increases normally with workload and reaches the predicted maximum (shaded area at the top).

Interpretation: For an overweight (body mass index = 30 kg/m^2) sedentary man, this is a 'normal' exercise test. He achieved a peak $\dot{V}O_2$ of 77% predicted when this is corrected for his body weight. His peak heart rate reached 78% of his predicted maximum, which is similar to his oxygen uptake. His breathing reserve is high (62%), confirming that his respiratory system is not limiting his exercise capacity. There is nothing in this test to indicate cardiovascular disease. His dyspnoea may be due to his obesity and lack of fitness, and he should address these issues.

Patient 9B: age 75, male, height 1.70 m, weight 62 kg

History: Ex-smoker of Asian origin. Presented with chest discomfort and subsequently found to have a potentially resectable bronchogenic carcinoma.

		Predicted	Measured	% predicted
Spirometry	FEV$_1$ litres	2.5	(1.42)	(57)
	FVC litres	3.8	2.53	67
	FEV$_1$/FVC %	68	56	
	FEF$_{25-75\%}$ L/s	2.29	0.51	22
Lung volumes	TLC litres	5.72	5.48	96
(plethysmograph)	RV litres	2.42	2.95	122
	RV/TLC %	42	54	
	FRC litres	3.62	3.44	95
	VC litres	3.80	2.53	67

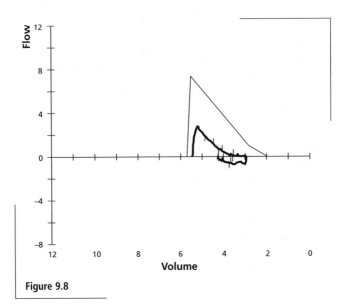

Figure 9.8

	Predicted	Measured	% predicted
Gas transfer			
DLco mL/min/mmHg	15.6	10.9	70
DLco/VA mL/min/mmHg/L	3.52	3.16	90
VA litres		3.46	

Interpretation: The results suggest a predominantly obstructive defect. The predicted values are based on Caucasians and, if they were corrected for this Asian man by a reduction of 10–12%, the lung volumes would be above normal and the RV would suggest gas trapping. The DLco is low/normal, but the 'normal' range is very broad in this age group. It would be consistent with undiagnosed emphysema. He was referred for exercise testing to assess his suitability for pulmonary resection.

Exercise report
Resting data: heart rate 95/min, $\dot{V}O_2$ 0.178 L/min, respiratory rate 22/min

The patient exercised on a treadmill for 4 minutes at a speed of 2 km/h. The slope was progressively increased by 2% each minute up to 6%. He stopped due to extreme dyspnoea.

On peak exertion

	Predicted	Measured	% predicted
Oxygen uptake			
$\dot{V}O_2$ mL/kg/min	18.8	(9.0)	(48)
$\dot{V}O_2$ L/min	1.80	(0.56)	(31)
Oxygen saturation		94%	
Cardiovascular response			
Heart rate beats/min	145	158	(109)
O_2 pulse mL/beat		3.5	
Ventilatory response			
Ventilation L/min	49.7*	25.5	51
Breathing reserve		49%	
Respiratory exchange ratio		0.98	
(*maximum ventilation predicted from $35 \times FEV_1$)			

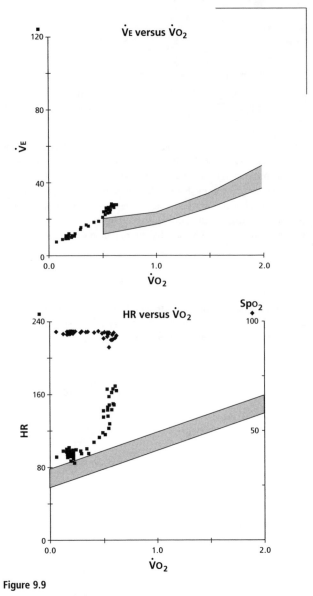

Figure 9.9

Interpretation: He achieved a very low level of exercise, reaching only 31% of his predicted maximum $\dot{V}O_2$. He had a high resting heart rate and numerous supraventricular and ventricular ectopic beats were noted. His respiratory rate was also high and both the heart and respiratory rate increased excessively with exercise. He stopped the exercise test because of dyspnoea and the question is whether his cardiovascular or respiratory system is limiting him. His breathing reserve at peak exercise is high (approximately 50%), but he has exceeded his predicted maximum heart rate. The oxygen pulse is very low (note that no predicted maximum value is provided because no reliable normal data are available for this age group, but we can estimate that it should be around 7.5 mL/beat from his predicted maximum $\dot{V}O_2$ divided by his predicted maximum heart rate).

The exercise test suggests that his poor exercise tolerance is principally due to his cardiovascular system. He had originally presented with chest pain, and further investigation revealed a severe left main coronary artery lesion. This was treated with angioplasty and stenting, and he subsequently proceeded to an uneventful resection of his lung cancer.

Patient 9C: age 42, female, height 1.65 m, weight 57.5 kg

History: Recent ex-smoker of 40 pack-years (1 pack-year is the equivalent of smoking 1 pack of 20 cigarettes a day for 1 year). Presents with rapidly progressive dyspnoea and chest tightness over 3–4 months.

		Predicted	Measured	% predicted
Spirometry	FEV$_1$ litres	2.8	2.59	92
	FVC litres	3.62	4.20	116
	FEV$_1$/FVC %	77	62	
	FEF$_{25-75\%}$ L/s	3.19	(1.36)	(43)
Lung volumes	TLC litres	5.24	(6.46)	(123)
(plethysmograph)	RV litres	1.76	2.26	128
	RV/TLC %	33	35	
	FRC litres	3.06	3.83	125
	VC litres	3.62	4.20	116

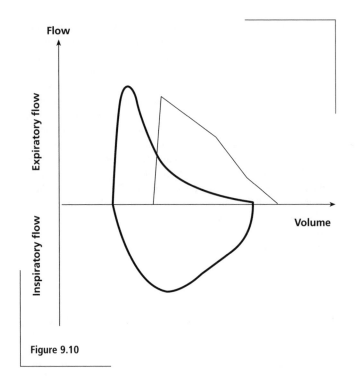

Figure 9.10

	Predicted	Measured	% predicted
Gas transfer			
DLco mL/min/mmHg	20.8	(5.5)	(27)
DLco/VA mL/min/mmHg/L	4.26	(1.06)	(25)
VA litres		5.20	

Interpretation: This is the same patient as Patient 2A. Lung volumes have now been added. She has evidence of mild obstructive airways disease on spirometry on the flow-volume loop. The lung volume is in the high/normal range. The most striking abnormality is the profound reduction in gas transfer which is out of keeping with the extent of her obstructive airways disease. An exercise test was performed.

Exercise report

Resting data: heart rate 87/min, $\dot{V}O_2$ 0.313 L/min, respiratory rate 20/min

The patient exercised on a treadmill for 3 minutes at a speed of 3 km/h. The slope was progressively increased by 2% each minute up to 4%. She stopped due to dyspnoea and a fall in oxygen saturation.

On peak exertion

	Predicted	Measured	% predicted
Oxygen uptake			
$\dot{V}O_2$ mL/kg/min	32.5	(12.7)	(39)
$\dot{V}O_2$ L/min	2.01	(0.73)	(36)
Oxygen saturation		80%	
Cardiovascular response			
Heart rate beats/min	172	121	(71)
O_2 pulse mL/beat	10.0	6.0	(61)
Ventilatory response			
Ventilation L/min	90.7*	57.1	63
Breathing reserve		37%	
Respiratory exchange ratio		0.90	
(*maximum ventilation predicted from $35 \times FEV_1$)			

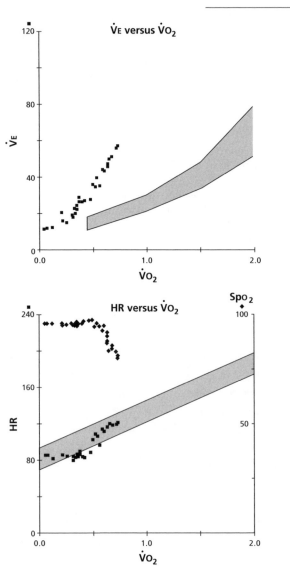

Figure 9.11

Interpretation: She has excessive ventilation from the start of exercise and only achieves 36% of her predicted maximum oxygen uptake. Her heart rate response and oxygen pulse responses are normal (she does not reach the predicted maximums because she stops exercising too early). The abrupt oxygen desaturation reflects her limited gas exchange (low DLCO). Her exercise capacity is limited by her respiratory system. In the absence of significant interstitial lung disease or major obstructive airways disease, this pattern would raise the suspicion of pulmonary hypertension. She did in fact have pulmonary hypertension of unknown cause.

Patient 9D: age 51, male, height 1.77 m, weight 90 kg

History: History of breathlessness and chest tightness for 1 year noticed on hiking with his wife. Ex-smoker, 18 pack-years, having stopped 12 years ago. Mild, well-controlled hypertension and strong family history of ischaemic heart disease—brother died of this at the age of 54. Denies other respiratory symptoms.

	Predicted	Measured	% predicted	After bronchodilator
Spirometry				
FEV$_1$ litres	3.55	3.14	88	3.35
FVC litres	4.84	5.23	108	5.47
FEV$_1$/FVC%	73	60		61
FEF$_{25-75\%}$ L/s	3.51	(1.41)	(40)	(1.62)
Lung volumes (plethysmograph)				
TLC litres	6.80	(8.78)	(129)	(8.70)
RV litres	2.22	(3.35)	(151)	(3.23)
RV/TLC %	34	38		37
FRC litres	3.60	(5.12)	(142)	4.57
VC litres	4.84	5.43	112	5.47
Gas transfer				
DLCO mL/min/mmHg	26.8		27.8	104
DLCO/VA mL/min/mmHg/L	4.12		3.93	96
VA litres			7.08	

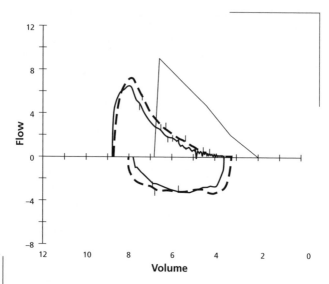

Figure 9.12
The broken line indicates the flow-volume loop after bronchodilator. Note that the inspiratory loops do not join up with the expiratory loops at TLC. This suggests either an air leak or incomplete inspiration (as in this case).

Interpretation: There is evidence of mild airflow obstruction with a reduced FEV_1/FVC ratio and an abnormal flow-volume loop. He has hyperinflation and gas trapping but normal gas transfer. There is no significant response to bronchodilator. In view of the cardiac history and the relatively normal FEV_1, an exercise test was performed.

Exercise report
Resting data: heart rate 93/min, $\dot{V}O_2$ 0.306 L/min, respiratory rate 20/min

The patient exercised on a treadmill for 8 minutes at a speed of 4 km/h. The slope was progressively increased by 2% each minute up to 14%. The test was stopped because the patient reached the predicted maximum heart rate.

On peak exertion

	Predicted	Measured	% predicted
Oxygen uptake			
$\dot{V}O_2$ mL/kg/min	32.0	26.9	84
$\dot{V}O_2$ L/min	2.57	2.42	94
Oxygen saturation		97%	
Cardiovascular response			
Heart rate beats/min	165	166	100
O_2 pulse mL/beat	16.5	14.6	88
Ventilatory response			
Ventilation L/min	109.9*	80.5	73
Breathing reserve		27%	
Respiratory exchange ratio		1.05	
(*maximum ventilation predicted from $35 \times FEV_1$)			

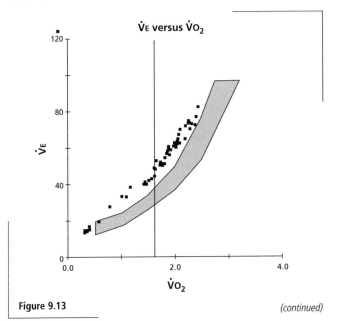

Figure 9.13

(continued)

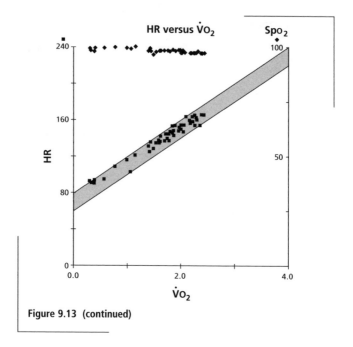

Figure 9.13 (continued)

Interpretation: He achieved a normal level of exercise and the test was stopped because he reached his predicted maximum heart rate. The cardiovascular responses to exercise were normal and there is no evidence of a cardiovascular limitation to exercise. Ventilation was slightly excessive at all levels of exercise but he was not limited by his respiratory system either, although he does have a slightly low breathing reserve of 27% (normal is 30–40%).

Patient 9E: age 42, male, height 1.77 m, weight 92.5 kg
History: Three-month history of rapidly progressive dyspnoea and a dry cough. Ex-smoker and has been exposed to a variety of chemicals and dusts in his occupation in a chemical works.

		Predicted	Measured	% predicted
Spirometry	FEV$_1$ litres	3.84	(1.49)	(49)
	FVC litres	5.07	(2.09)	(41)
	FEV$_1$/FVC %	75	71	
	FEF$_{25-75\%}$ L/s	3.91	(1.00)	(26)
Lung volumes	TLC litres	6.93	(3.53)	(51)
(plethysmograph)	RV litres	2.07	1.40	68
	RV/TLC %	31	40	
	FRC litres	3.55	(2.11)	(59)
	VC litres	5.07	(2.13)	(42)
Gas transfer				
	DLco mL/min/mmHg	29.3	(20.3)	(69)
	DLco/VA mL/min/mmHg/L	4.31	5.99	139
	VA litres		3.38	

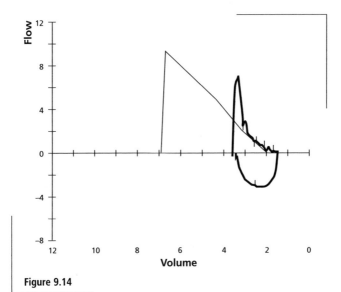

Figure 9.14

Interpretation: He has a severe restrictive defect. Gas transfer is impaired, but this corrects for lung volume (DLco/VA or Kco). He underwent progressive exercise testing.

Exercise report
Resting data: heart rate 80/min, $\dot{V}O_2$ 0.364 L/min, respiratory rate 17/min

The patient exercised on a treadmill for 6 minutes at a speed of 4 km/h. The slope was progressively increased by 2% each minute up to 10%. The test was stopped because of dyspnoea and because the oxygen saturation fell.

On peak exertion

	Predicted	Measured	% predicted
Oxygen uptake			
$\dot{V}O_2$ mL/kg/min	36.9	(20.0)	(54)
$\dot{V}O_2$ L/min	2.86	(1.85)	(65)
Oxygen saturation		81%	
Cardiovascular response			
Heart rate beats/min	172	127	74
O_2 pulse mL/beat	16.5	14.6	88
Ventilatory response			
Ventilation L/min	52.2*	55.9	107
Breathing reserve		−7%	
Respiratory exchange ratio		0.98	
(*maximum ventilation predicted from 35 × FEV_1)			

Interpretation: He achieved a surprisingly high workload, achieving a peak oxygen uptake of 65% predicted. Ventilation was excessive throughout the test but this failed to prevent a fall in oxygen saturation. The cardiovascular responses to exercise were normal and there is no evidence of a cardiovascular limitation to exercise. The breathing reserve is very low (−7%: he exceeded his maximum predicted ventilation) and this indicates that the limitation to exercise is respiratory in origin.

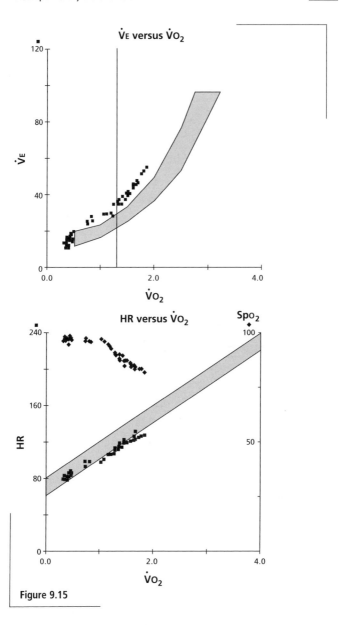

Figure 9.15

Further investigation of this patient confirmed that he had fibrosing alveolitis (idiopathic pulmonary fibrosis). He continued to deteriorate symptomatically despite treatment, and pulmonary function and exercise tests were repeated 11 and 15 months after his initial evaluation.

		Initial	11 months	15 months
Spirometry	FEV$_1$ litres	1.49	1.53	1.40
	FVC litres	2.09	2.08	1.76
	FEV$_1$/FVC %	71	74	80
	FEF$_{25-75\%}$ L/s	1.00	1.08	1.32
Lung volumes	TLC litres	3.53	3.29	2.99
	RV litres	1.40	1.16	1.24
	RV/TLC %	40	35	41
	FRC litres	2.11	1.78	1.94
	VC litres	2.13	2.13	1.76
Gas transfer				
	DLco mL/min/mmHg	20.3	13.8	11.0
	DLco/VA mL/min/mmHg/L	5.99	5.17	4.58
	VA litres	3.38	2.67	2.39
Peak exercise responses				
	$\dot{V}o_2$ mL/kg/min	20.0	18.3	12.0
	$\dot{V}o_2$ L/min	1.85	1.74	1.14
	Oxygen saturation	81%	79%	79%
	Heart rate beats/min	127	129	112
	O$_2$ pulse mL/beat	14.6	13.5	10.1
	Ventilation L/min	55.9	63.8	47.0

Interpretation: His lung function tests show a progressive decline despite treatment. The spirometric values become more 'restrictive', the lung volume falls and the gas transfer becomes severely impaired. His exercise tolerance falls (he managed 6 minutes on the first test, 5 minutes on the second, but only 1 minute 40 seconds on the final test). As there was a progressive decline with no response to therapy, the patient was put on the waiting list for lung transplantation.

Patient 9F: age 76, male, height 1.77 m, weight 79 kg

History: Presents with exertional dyspnoea for 1 year. Ex-smoker of 30 pack-years, stopped 15 years ago. No other respiratory symptoms.

		Predicted	Measured	% predicted
Spirometry	FEV$_1$ litres	2.75	2.38	87
	FVC litres	4.22	3.21	76
	FEV$_1$/FVC %	67	74	
	FEF$_{25-75\%}$ L/s	2.38	1.63	68
Lung volumes	TLC litres	6.42	5.80	90
(plethysmograph)	RV litres	2.64	2.60	98
	RV/TLC %	43	45	
	FRC litres	3.80	3.41	90
	VC litres	4.22	3.21	76
Gas transfer				
DL$_{CO}$ mL/min/mmHg		19.1	13.4	70
DL$_{CO}$/VA mL/min/mmHg/L		3.49	2.88	82
VA litres			4.65	

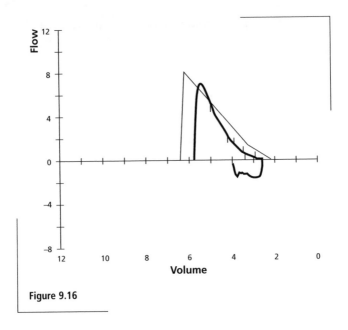

Figure 9.16

Interpretation: The spirometry data would be compatible with a slight restrictive defect, but there is no hard evidence for this and the TLC is well within the normal range. Gas transfer is also at the lower end of the normal range (which is quite broad in this age group). He was investigated further with a progressive exercise test.

Exercise report
Resting data: heart rate 62/min, $\dot{V}O_2$ 0.240 L/min, respiratory rate 18/min

The patient exercised on a treadmill for 7 minutes at a speed of 4 km/h. The slope was progressively increased by 2% each minute up to 12%. The test was stopped because the patient became short of breath.

On peak exertion

	Predicted	Measured	% predicted
Oxygen uptake			
$\dot{V}o_2$ mL/kg/min	18.2	16.1	(88)
$\dot{V}o_2$ L/min	1.77	(1.27)	(72)
Oxygen saturation		71%	
Cardiovascular response			
Heart rate beats/min	135	98	73
O_2 pulse mL/beat		12.9	
Ventilatory response			
Ventilation L/min	83.3*	48.2	58
Breathing reserve		42%	
Respiratory exchange ratio		1.12	

(*maximum ventilation predicted from $35 \times FEV_1$)

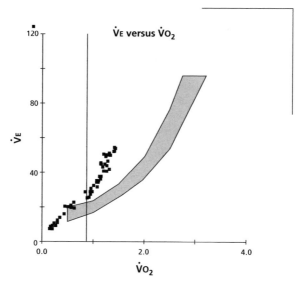

Figure 9.17

(continued)

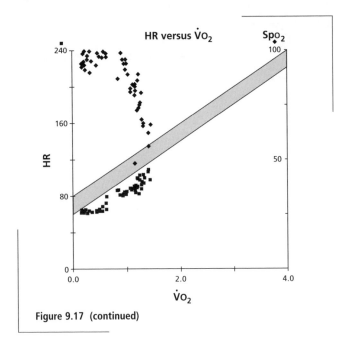

Figure 9.17 (continued)

Interpretation: He had severe oxygen desaturation during exercise. Despite this his peak oxygen uptake was only slightly reduced. His ventilatory response was excessive. The cardiovascular response was normal (there is no predicted 'normal' for oxygen pulse for a man of this age but it is estimated to be approximately 13 mL/beat). The breathing reserve is normal, but the exercise test still suggests a respiratory limitation to exercise.

He was investigated further with a high-resolution CT scan which revealed pulmonary fibrosis suggestive of cryptogenic fibrosing alveolitis (idiopathic pulmonary fibrosis).

Chapter 10

Exhaled nitric oxide

Measurement of exhaled nitric oxide (eNO) is a recent addition to many lung function laboratories. High levels of eNO are typically found in patients with asthma and appear to indicate airway inflammation. Measurement of eNO complements traditional tests of airway function such as spirometry and bronchial responsiveness, and is developing a role in the diagnosis and management of asthma. Although airway and alveolar inflammation occurs in many other respiratory diseases, the role of eNO in diagnosing and managing these conditions remains unclear.

Measuring eNO

Nitric oxide is present in exhaled air in trace amounts only—a few parts per billion—and it requires a very sensitive (and usually expensive) analyser to measure this. A number of techniques have been described, including collecting samples of exhaled air for analysis offline. Most laboratories measure nitric oxide online while the patient exhales at a constant flow through the analyser. The procedure is quite easy and most patients are able to provide satisfactory tests after a few practices to get the right flow rate.

The procedure is generally as follows:
- The patient inhales maximally through their mouth (to TLC).
- On reaching full inspiration, the patient immediately breathes out through a mouthpiece against a resistance.

- A biofeedback device indicates whether the patient is breathing out too slowly or too quickly. The patient adjusts the speed of exhalation accordingly.
- The analyser measures the exhaled nitric oxide level throughout the procedure.
- The patient continues until full expiration, or until a satisfactory plateau has been reached on the eNO curve.
- The procedure is repeated until two or three satisfactory exhalations have been recorded. These should be repeatable to within 10%.
- A plateau is generally defined as a three-second period during which there is less than 10% variation in the nitric oxide level. This can sometimes be hard to achieve or recognise.

The most important issues are the exhalation flow rate and avoiding contamination of the exhaled air with air from the nose.

The exhalation flow rate is important because it affects the concentration of eNO—the faster the flow, the lower the eNO. Alveolar air contains very little nitric oxide (it is taken up by haemoglobin in pulmonary capillaries) and hence the nitric oxide in exhaled air originates in the upper and lower airways. The slower we exhale, the more time there is for nitric oxide to diffuse from the airway wall into the exhaled air. This makes a big difference to the measurement—eNO measured at 50 mL/sec is more than two times higher than eNO measured at 250 mL/sec. At the moment there appears to be little to choose between different flows. At low flows there is more nitric oxide to measure but the results may be more variable. Current recommendations suggest a flow of 50 mL/sec, but 250 mL/sec has also been widely used, and higher and lower flows may be just as good. Whichever flow is used, it should be reported with the test result.

Avoiding contamination with nasal air is important because the concentration of nitric oxide in the nose is many times higher than in the bronchi. Most techniques prevent nasal nitric oxide from mixing with the exhaled air by getting the patient to exhale against a resistance. This creates a pressure in the oropharynx that is sufficient to raise the soft palate and close the posterior nasopharynx. (The level of *nasal* nitric oxide can also be measured. The clinical usefulness of this is uncertain, except for the rare disorder of primary ciliary dyskinesia, in which nasal nitric oxide is much lower than normal.)

The concentration of nitric oxide in ambient air varies substantially and may be higher than the concentration in exhaled air. Although this appears to have little impact on the level of nitric oxide in exhaled air, it may cause a high peak in the eNO curve, and occasionally patients are unable to exhale for long enough for the curve to reach a plateau. Some protocols require the patient to inhale nitric oxide-free air before exhaling into the analyser. It is recommended that the ambient level be stated on the report. Similarly, inhalation through the nose will cause an initial peak in the eNO curve (because of the very high concentration of nitric oxide in the nose) and patients should be encouraged to inhale through their mouth. Breath holding at the end of full inspiration, before exhalation through the analyser, can allow nitric oxide to build up in the upper airways and cause an early peak, and this should be avoided.

A number of other factors may affect eNO levels. The influence of other lung function tests on eNO is uncertain and it is recommended that eNO measurement be done first. Smoking is known to reduce eNO and patients should avoid smoking for at least an hour before the test. eNO may also be reduced in chronic cigarette smokers and smoking history should be noted. Some foods may alter nitric oxide production, and eating and drinking should be avoided for two hours before the test. Viral respiratory infections are thought to increase eNO levels, whereas HIV infection is associated with reduced eNO levels. Drugs may also alter eNO levels—particularly asthma medications such as inhaled corticosteroids (one of the roles of eNO measurement is to monitor the effect of anti-inflammatory asthma treatments). Bronchodilators may alter eNO levels indirectly by changing airway calibre.

Many potential influences on eNO measurement have not been explored. Even the influences of age and sex are not fully described. eNO has been reported to vary throughout the menstrual cycle. Perhaps because of these issues and the continuing uncertainty regarding the optimal measurement technique, there are no widely recognised prediction equations for eNO. Until these have been developed, each laboratory should define its own normal values and specify the population to whom the values apply.

Interpreting eNO

eNO is primarily used to diagnose and monitor asthma. Although other conditions may be associated with altered levels of eNO, the alterations in these conditions are generally less extreme than in asthma and it is not clear whether eNO measurement has any role in their management.

In a patient suspected of having asthma, a high eNO strongly supports the diagnosis. Measuring eNO appears to be as good a diagnostic test for asthma as bronchial challenge techniques and has the advantage of being quicker and simpler to perform. In a patient known to have asthma, a high eNO suggests poorly controlled airway inflammation. The eNO level may be monitored to adjust the dose of inhaled corticosteroid treatment.

More work needs to be done on the following uses of eNO:

- whether it can effectively distinguish asthma from COPD and other causes of airflow obstruction
- whether it can be used to predict which patients with other diseases (such as COPD) will respond to anti-inflammatory treatment (such as inhaled corticosteroids)
- its utility in monitoring asthma control.

We can expect changes in the measurement techniques and interpretation of eNO in the future.

For more information see 'ATS/ERS recommendations for standardized procedures for the online and offline measurement of exhaled lower respiratory nitric oxide and nasal nitric oxide', *American Journal of Respiratory and Critical Care Medicine*, 2005, 171, pp. 912–30.

Other techniques to measure airway inflammation

There has been much interest in non-invasive techniques to measure airway inflammation. To date, only eNO is widely used for clinical purposes. *Induced sputum analysis* can be very informative, but it is time-consuming to perform and requires specialised laboratory skills. Hence it is still mostly used for research. *Exhaled breath condensate* analysis is a recent development. It involves collecting moisture condensed from exhaled breath over a few minutes. This has been found to contain trace amounts of airway chemicals. A wide variety of substances, from pH to inflammatory cytokines, have been analysed and linked to airway diseases. The technique appears to be promising, but at present it remains a research tool.

CHAPTER SUMMARY

→ Exhaled nitric oxide (eNO) is a simple, non-invasive test of airway inflammation.
→ A raised nitric oxide supports a clinical diagnosis of asthma and may be useful for monitoring the response to treatment.
→ The role of nitric oxide measurement in the management and diagnosis of other diseases is uncertain.

. . . see over for a clinical example

Clinical example

Patient 10A: age 31, male, height 1.80 m, weight 97 kg

History: Shortness of breath associated with wheeze on exertion 'for as long as he can remember'. Has never been diagnosed as having asthma and has never tried any asthma treatment. History of hay fever. Has never smoked.

	Predicted	Measured	% predicted
FEV$_1$ litres	4.61	4.49	97
FVC litres	5.58	6.25	112
FEV$_1$/FVC %	83	72	

Spirometry was repeated 15 minutes after bronchodilator.

	Measured	% predicted	% change
FEV$_1$ litres	4.71	102	5
FVC litres	6.24	112	0
FEV$_1$/FVC %	75		

eNO measured at 50 mL/s (measured before spirometry) = 76.5 ppb

Ambient NO level = 2.3 ppb

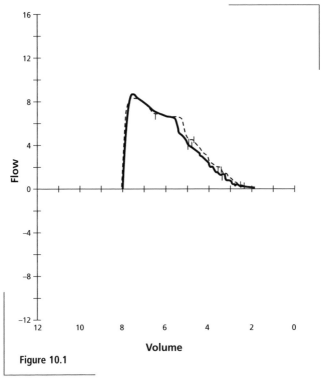

Figure 10.1

Interpretation: The pre-bronchodilator FEV_1 and FVC are both within normal limits, although the FEV_1/FVC ratio is lower than expected, which is compatible with mild airflow obstruction. The 320 mL increase in the FEV_1 after bronchodilator is not significant according to reversibility criteria because this is only a 5% change. The flow-volume loop shows a 'knee' but no evidence of obstruction. The eNO is high—95% of non-asthmatic adult males in this laboratory have an eNO below 45 ppb.

Is this asthma? Probably. The patient has exercise symptoms suggestive of asthma and evidence of airway inflammation. However, there is scant evidence of airflow obstruction and little response to bronchodilator. The diagnosis has not been confirmed by the traditional lung function criteria. It may be worth performing a bronchial challenge. An alternative approach would be to treat the airway inflammation to see whether the symptoms and spirometry improve.

Chapter 11

Miscellaneous tests

Airway resistance/conductance

Another method of assessing airway calibre uses *airway resistance* (Raw). This is usually done in a plethysmograph in which the difference in pressure inside the box and inside the chest can be measured at the same time as airflow at the mouth (see *Raw and SGaw*). These measurements can be used to calculate the airways' resistance to airflow (Raw). Airway conductance (Gaw) is the reciprocal of resistance and is another way of presenting the same information. Resistance to airflow varies at different lung volumes because airways are wider at high lung volumes than at low lung volumes. Raw is therefore normally measured at FRC to standardise the measurement. Another way of standardising the measurement is to multiply or divide the measurement by the lung volume at which it was measured to calculate the specific airway resistance (SRaw) or specific airway conductance (SGaw) respectively.

Airway resistance is a sensitive way of detecting airflow obstruction. It may detect early disease before this becomes apparent on spirometry. However, its measurement in the body box is prone to a number of errors. The calculations involved in deriving Raw may compound these errors. Most laboratories measure Raw on inspiration and may underestimate obstruction in patients with emphysema and airways collapse on expiration. It is generally regarded as less reliable than spirometry and adds little to the evaluation of most patients. However, it may be useful in patients who are unable or

Raw AND SGaw

Airway resistance and specific airway conductance are often measured at the same time as lung volumes in the body box. When the patient pants with the shutter open, the airflow through the mouthpiece is measured by a flow sensor (pneumotachograph). This flow can be related to the small pressure changes in the box. The patient continues to pant while the shutter is closed. When the shutter is closed, there is no flow and the measured mouth pressure equals the alveolar pressure. Changes in mouth pressure can be related to the fluctuation in box pressure. Combining the ratios of *flow:box pressure* and *alveolar pressure:box pressure* allows the *pressure:flow* relationship of the airways to be calculated.

Airway resistance (Raw) is the pressure required (alveolar to mouth) to generate a unit of airflow through the airways.

Airway conductance (Gaw) is the reciprocal of Raw—the airflow generated per unit of pressure. Because the conductance of the airways increases with lung volume, *specific airway conductance* (SGaw), which is the conductance divided by the VTG at which the measurements were made, is usually reported.

unwilling to perform maximal expiratory manoeuvres. It is less effort-dependent than spirometry but does require coordination and some patients may be unable to produce satisfactory measurements. Raw is usually measured at the same time as lung volumes in the body plethysmograph and is often included in the report.

Forced oscillation techniques

The principles of the forced oscillation technique (FOT) were developed 50 years ago but technical requirements prevented its widespread use. However, commercial systems based on this technique have recently been developed, including the *random oscillatory system* and the *impulse oscillation system*. These systems are becoming widely available, meaning that FOT is now feasible as a routine measurement in many respiratory laboratories. The different systems apply the same basic concepts but differ in the shape and frequencies of the oscillating signal and in their method of analysing the data. The relative merits of each system have not been established.

Forced oscillation techniques have the potential to address two limitations in our ability to measure lung function:

1. Many children under 10 and some adults are incapable of carrying out repeatable and technically adequate spirometry, leading to difficulties in diagnosis and treatment in these patients. Forced oscillation technique measurements are possible in these groups, allowing assessment of lung function.

2. Standard spirometry and airways resistance measurements in the body box do not distinguish small airways disease from large airways disease. Theoretically, forced oscillation techniques can partition the airways resistance and airways reactance measurements into peripheral and central airway components. Whether this is clinically useful remains to be seen.

The technique works by 'forcing' small amplitude vibrating or oscillating signals of varying frequency from a loudspeaker into the airway during tidal breathing. The effect of this signal on the oscillatory flow signals is determined by the mechanical properties of the respiratory system. The technique is very easy for patients to perform. The only cooperation required is to breathe normally through an airtight mouthpiece while wearing a nose clip. To the patient, the forced oscillating signals feel like a light tapping on the mouthpiece. The normal pattern of these measurements is shown in Figure 11.1.

Multiple oscillations are made during the breathing cycle. Measurements made when the oscillations are in phase with airflow measure respiratory resistance (Rrs), and respiratory reactance (Xrs) is measured when the oscillations are out of phase with airflow. Respiratory reactance reflects both the impedance and the elastance of the respiratory system. In theory, low-frequency oscillations measure resistance and reactance of the peripheral airways and high-frequency oscillations measure the central airways. In early obstructive disease, airways changes in respiratory resistance (Rrs) may be detectable when spirometry is still normal.

Interpretation of the results remains a problem. Neither of the currently available commercial systems gives a coherence value—a measure of the reproducibility of the signal at each frequency. Population-based reference values for adults are not yet available and data sets in children are only just beginning to appear. However, pattern recognition can point to problems. Serial random oscillatory system data from a patient undergoing lung transplantation are

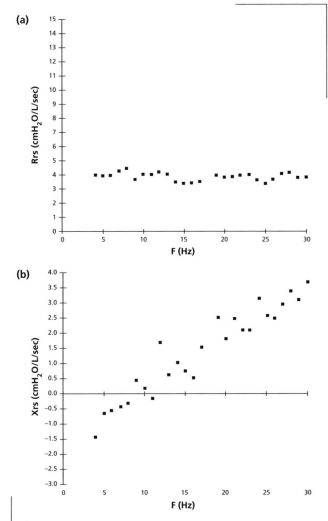

Figure 11.1
(a) The normal pattern of respiratory resistance measurements (Rrs) across the range of frequencies (F(Hz)) in an individual with normal lung function.
(b) The pattern of reactance measurements (Xrs) across the frequency range (F(Hz)) in the same individual.

demonstrated. Figure 11.2 shows serial respiratory resistance measurements Rrs or Zr (different systems use different nomenclature), and in Figure 11.3 serial respiratory reactance measurements Xrs or Zi are shown.

This technique is showing promise in research examining the effect of interventions on pulmonary mechanics (e.g. bronchial challenge testing or the response to bronchodilating drugs). This method is able to detect treatment-related changes and can potentially localise the site of these changes to the central or peripheral airways.

For further reading on the theory behind this technique and its clinical applications see ERS Task Force, 'The forced oscillation technique in clinical practice: methodology, recommendations and future developments', *European Respiratory Journal*, 2003, 22, pp. 1026–41.

Lung compliance

An alternative way of measuring intrathoracic pressure is to use an oesophageal balloon. This can be used to measure lung compliance (C_L). *Lung compliance* is defined as the change in lung volume for a given change in elastic recoil pressure. Because of their elasticity, the lungs try to collapse. This is counterbalanced by the chest wall which tries to expand, creating a negative intrapleural pressure. This negative pressure is increased at high lung volumes because of increased stretching of the lungs. The change in lung volume (measured by a spirometer at the mouth) for a change in pressure (measured by the oesophageal balloon) is used to calculate the compliance. *Static lung compliance* (C_{Lstat}) is calculated by measuring the pressure when there is no airflow at two different lung volumes. Compliance decreases in fibrotic lung diseases, which stiffen the lungs, and increases in emphysema, in which the lungs are floppy. *Dynamic lung compliance* (C_{Ldyn}) is measured during tidal breathing by continuously measuring volume and pressure, then measuring the slope of the line joining the points when airflow ceases at each end of the respiratory cycle. Dynamic compliance is similar to the respective static compliance in normal and fibrotic lungs, but in patients with peripheral airways disease C_{Ldyn} may be lower and varies with the frequency of breathing because of the uneven distribution of ventilation. While this can be used to detect early airways disease, it has not found its way into routine use.

Total thoracic compliance is sometimes measured in intubated and ventilated patients. The change in lung volume for a given change in

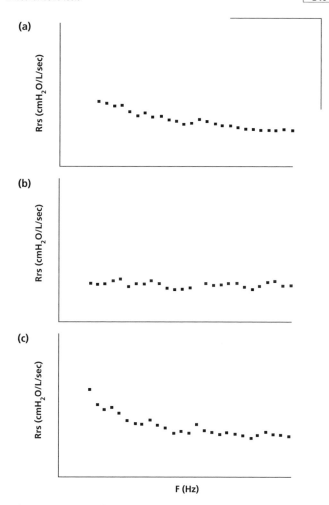

Figure 11.2 ROS resistance measurements (Rrs) in a woman with advanced emphysema, FEV$_1$ 19% predicted
(a) Prior to transplantation, illustrating high resistance at low frequencies. (b) Following lung transplantation (FEV$_1$ 89% predicted) the resistance pattern is normal. (c) Following development of bronchiolitis obliterans (chronic rejection) which destroys small airways (FEV$_1$ 43%), the resistance measurements at low frequencies increases again.

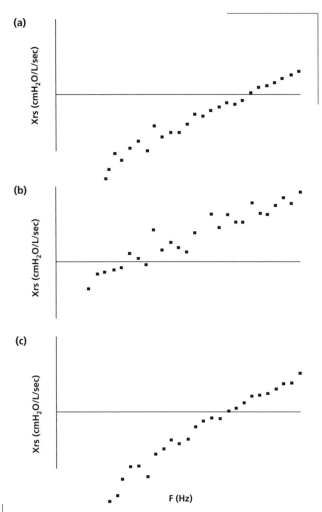

Figure 11.3 ROS reactance measurements (Xrs) in the same patient with advanced emphysema as shown in Figure 11.2

(a) Prior to lung transplantation, with low reactance measurements at low frequencies. (b) A normal reactance pattern following transplantation. (c) The recurrence of the low reactance measurements at low frequencies as bronchiolitis obliterans (chronic rejection) destroys small airways.

airway pressure can be measured from the ventilator circuit. It requires the respiratory muscles to be relaxed, usually with neuromuscular blocking agents. It reflects both lung compliance and the compliance of the chest wall and may be altered by diseases of either. Adult respiratory distress syndrome causes the lungs to stiffen and decreases compliance.

Nitrogen washout tests

A number of nitrogen washout tests can be used to calculate lung volumes and to detect uneven ventilation. In the *multiple-breath nitrogen washout* technique, the patient breathes 100% oxygen for 7 minutes. The exhaled gas is analysed breath by breath along with the tidal volume (or collected in a bag and its nitrogen concentration analysed). The concentration of nitrogen in the exhaled gas falls as nitrogen is replaced by oxygen. In normal patients the nitrogen should be washed out of the lungs in 3–4 minutes and the concentration in the exhaled air at the end of the test should be less than 1.5%. Since the volume of nitrogen exhaled and the starting concentration of nitrogen in the lung (approximately 80%) have been measured, the volume of gas in the thorax can be calculated (small adjustments are necessary to allow for nitrogen diffusing out of blood and tissue, and the concentration of nitrogen in the exhaled air at the end of the test). This method will underestimate the lung volumes if there is air trapped in bullae for the same reason as in the helium dilution technique.

Failure of the concentration of nitrogen to fall below 2.5% after 7 minutes of breathing pure oxygen suggests uneven ventilation (characteristic of all obstructive diseases). Uneven ventilation may also be detected if the concentration of nitrogen in each breath is plotted against the volume exhaled. If the distribution of ventilation is even, this will appear as a straight line. If there is uneven distribution or gas trapping, the curve will be concave.

The *single-breath nitrogen washout test* involves the subject inhaling 100% oxygen in a single breath from residual volume up to total lung capacity. The subject then carries out a slow steady maximal exhalation. During the exhalation the concentration of exhaled nitrogen is measured continuously and plotted against expired volume.

The resultant curve can be divided into a series of phases (Fig. 11.4):

• Phase I—no nitrogen is detected as anatomical dead space (pharynx, trachea, bronchi) is emptied.

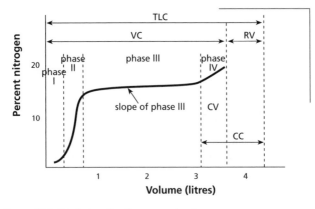

Figure 11.4 Single-breath nitrogen washout curve

- Phase II—in this phase there is a rapid rise in nitrogen concentration as alveoli start to empty and mix with the remaining anatomical dead-space gas (pure oxygen).
- Phase III—in this phase the slope is much flatter as alveolar emptying continues. The slope of this phase is measured to determine the uniformity of ventilation. It is approximately 1–1.5% (change in nitrogen concentration per litre) in healthy young adults and up to 3% in the elderly. In airways disease the slope tends to be much steeper due to uneven emptying.
- Phase IV—at this point the slope abruptly increases due to airway narrowing or closure in the dependent parts of the lung, and so more of the expired gas is coming from the upper lobes. Because these alveoli are relatively well-inflated even at residual volume (the effect of gravity tends to compress the basal alveoli but stretch the upper alveoli), less oxygen has entered them, resulting in a higher nitrogen concentration. The lung volume of phase IV (from the onset of phase IV to residual volume) is the closing volume (CV). In health this is usually less than 20% of the vital capacity. The closing capacity (CC) is the closing volume plus the residual volume. The CC is usually less than 30% of the total lung capacity. Increases in the CV or CC may indicate small airways disease, but there is a wide range of normal values. Restrictive diseases may also increase the ratio of the CV to the vital capacity and of the CC relative to the TLC by reducing the vital capacity and TLC.

The single-breath nitrogen washout test is relatively simple technically and has been used in epidemiological studies, but lack of good
data on normal values and both sensitivity and specificity have limited its widespread application.

Maximum voluntary ventilation

The maximum voluntary ventilation (MVV) is occasionally measured
by asking the patient to breathe as hard and as fast as possible for
12–15 seconds and extrapolating the volume to 1 minute. It is a non-
specific test and the MMV can be reduced in obstructive or restrictive
disorders. However, it is more sensitive to airflow obstruction and
may show normal values in some patients with restriction. The MVV
can also be estimated by multiplying the FEV_1 by 35. If the measured
MVV is very different from this, the difference is likely to be due to
poor patient effort. Muscular weakness and large airways disease can
also cause a reduction in the MVV out of proportion to the FEV_1.

The MVV is useful in interpreting exercise tests. Healthy subjects
do not reach their MVV during exercise unless they are extremely
well-trained. Patients with obstructive disorders may reach their
MVV during exercise and this suggests a ventilatory limit to exercise
(see Chapter 9).

CHAPTER SUMMARY

→ SGaw and Raw are sensitive measures of airflow obstruction, but
   are prone to measurement error.
→ Forced oscillation techniques (ROS/IOS) are becoming
   increasingly available and may be useful for measuring lung
   function in children and adults who are unable to perform
   spirometry. Once reference sets are available then the role and
   applicability of these tests will become clearer.
→ Lung compliance is decreased in lung fibrosis and increased in
   emphysema. It is not often measured because of the need to
   place an oesophageal balloon.
→ Nitrogen washout techniques can be used to detect uneven
   distribution of ventilation, which may indicate early small
   airways disease.

Chapter 12

Assessing patients for thoracic resection

A common use of lung function tests is to assess whether a patient is fit for surgery. This is a particular problem when the planned surgery involves removal of lung tissue, since these patients often have poor lung function. This is a complex and controversial area as there is no simple test which will predict postoperative outcome. The issue is to identify not just the patients who are unlikely to survive surgery, but also those whose lung function and exercise capacity will be so reduced that their quality of life and/or life expectancy will be severely impaired. Many of these patients have lung cancer, and the desire to avoid postoperative mortality or morbidity has to be balanced against the fact that, for the vast majority of patients, surgery is their only chance of cure.

One approach is simply to walk the patient up several flights of stairs and thus judge their general fitness and their respiratory reserve. The ability to climb three flights of stairs has a high predictive value for an uncomplicated surgical course for a single lobectomy (five flights for removal of a whole lung (pneumonectomy)). However, stair climbing tests are difficult to standardise and, in patients unable to achieve the target, the criteria are not defined and are largely subjective.

An alternative approach is to use static lung function tests and predict the postoperative lung function that would follow the planned resection. Thus a right upper lobectomy would remove 3 of the 19 lung segments leaving 16/19 of the preoperative lung function. Surgery that will leave patients with more than 40% of their predicted FEV_1 and DLCO is likely to be tolerated. This approach assumes that all segments are equal. In fact, the lung to be removed could vary from a fully functioning segment to a collapsed, non-functioning area, the removal of which would have minimal functional impact. Quantitative ventilation/perfusion scanning has been developed to assess the contribution of the area of lung in question to the overall lung function. This has not found wide acceptance because of the overlap of lobes in standard nuclear medicine scanning images and the limited number of reports on the specificity of this technique. There is also evidence that predicting postoperative lung function based on preoperative tests may overestimate the eventual functional loss. There is some capacity for recovery and the long-term consequences of a lobectomy are usually small, while a pneumonectomy leads to a loss of about 33% in lung function tests and 20% in exercise tolerance.

Preoperative assessment based on lung function alone also has the limitation that it does not assess other major comorbidity, especially cardiac disease or the influence of malnutrition on postoperative complication rates. This has led to the use of exercise testing. Exercise tests are highly sensitive for patients with limited exercise capacity. They can also reveal unrecognised cardiac disease, which is common in this patient population. Unfortunately the specificity is low and the recognition of patients limited by lack of effort or deconditioning can be difficult. At best, exercise tests divide patients into low risk, medium risk and high risk groups. The risks increase as the maximum oxygen uptake ($\dot{V}o_2$max/kg) falls (see Table 12.1).

The issue of preoperative testing for lung resection has been brought into question by the development of lung volume reduction surgery for advanced emphysema in recent years. These patients often have end-stage emphysema and would not be accepted for resectional thoracic surgery for lung cancer on 'existing criteria' by many surgical units. Yet 5–15% of such patients undergoing lung volume reduction surgery have either established bronchial carcinoma or carcinoma-in-situ, as an incidental finding, in the resected lung tissue. These patients often have complicated postoperative courses but the vast majority make a full recovery from surgery. As a result of this experience, there is an increasing reluctance to be too dogmatic in the use of selection criteria for thoracic resection (see the recent guidelines in British Thoracic Society and Society of Cardiothoracic Surgeons of Great Britain and Ireland Working Party, 'Guidelines on the selection of patients with lung cancer for surgery', *Thorax*, 2001, 56(2), pp. 89–108, or the British Thoracic Society website, www. brit-thoracic.org.uk).

The final decision should be an individual one for each patient. Coexistent cardiac disease will demand a higher level of lung function postoperatively than a normal cardiovascular system does. To add to the uncertainty there is some evidence that the functional consequences of lobectomy can vary from minimal in most patients to major effects similar to pneumonectomy.

Table 12.1	Risk of thoracic surgery based on exercise capacity. This is a rough guide only and individual decision making cannot be emphasised enough. The divisions are arbitrary and risk should be viewed as a continuum. The predicted postoperative value should be taken into account, as well as the absolute preoperative values. A lower limit of 35% of the predicted $\dot{V}o_2$max has been suggested for safe resection.

$\dot{V}o_2$max (mL/kg/min)	Risk	Comment
>20	Low	Very low perioperative mortality and low postoperative morbidity.
15–20	Moderate	Relatively low risk of perioperative mortality but increased though largely acceptable risk of postoperative morbidity.
10–15	High	Very significantly increased risk of both perioperative mortality and postoperative morbidity, with risk compounded by the extent of resection (e.g. risk in pneumonectomy > risk in segmentectomy)
<10	Very high	Very high and probably unacceptable risk for major thoracic surgery.

CHAPTER SUMMARY

→ Lung function and exercise test results are only a guide to suitability for resection and must be correlated with the individual patient's clinical situation.

→ The aim is to help maximise the number of patients who successfully have their lung cancer resected while minimising perioperative deaths and unacceptable morbidity from the effects of lung resection on cardiorespiratory function.

. . . see over for a clinical example

Clinical example

Patient 12A: age 71, male, height 1.63 m, weight 63 kg

History: Presents with a 6-week history of haemoptysis, increased cough and dyspnoea. Heavy smoker. Long history of mild exertional dyspnoea and recurrent winter bronchitis. Chest X-ray showed a partial collapse of the right upper lobe, and an adenocarcinoma obstructing the right upper lobe bronchial orifice was found at bronchoscopy.

		Predicted	Measured	% predicted
Spirometry	FEV$_1$ litres	2.36	(0.68)	(29)
	FVC litres	3.46	(1.76)	(51)
	FEV$_1$/FVC %	70	39	
	FEF$_{25-75\%}$ L/s	2.33	(0.22)	(9)
Lung volumes	TLC litres	5.06	(7.23)	(143)
(plethysmograph)	RV litres	2.15	(5.47)	(255)
	RV/TLC %	41	76	
	FRC litres	3.07	(5.96)	(194)
	VC litres	3.46	(1.76)	(51)
Gas transfer				
	DLco mL/min/mmHg	15.9	14.4	91
	DLco/VA mL/min/mmHg/L	3.56	4.28	120
	VA litres		3.37	

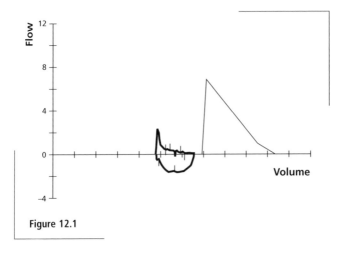

Figure 12.1

Interpretation: He has severe obstructive airways disease, with a very low FEV_1/FVC ratio, an abnormal flow-volume loop, hyperinflation and gas trapping. Gas transfer is surprisingly normal. He was insistent on a surgical assessment of his lung cancer, claiming that he had not been significantly limited by dyspnoea until the past 4 weeks. Although the tumour in the right upper lobe may be causing obstruction, the overall pattern of the test results suggests that he has a much more widespread abnormality. Progressive exercise testing was performed to further assess his suitability for surgical resection of his tumour.

Exercise report

Resting data: heart rate 102/min, $\dot{V}O_2$ 0.254 L/min, respiratory rate 19/min

The patient exercised on a treadmill for 7 minutes at a speed of 4 km/h. The slope was progressively increased by 2% each minute up to 12%. The test was stopped because the patient became uncomfortable.

On peak exertion

	Predicted	Measured	% predicted
Oxygen uptake			
$\dot{V}O_2$ mL/kg/min	21.0	(13.7)	(65)
$\dot{V}O_2$ L/min	1.93	(0.86)	(45)
Oxygen saturation %		91	
Cardiovascular response			
Heart rate beats/min	149	132	88
O_2 pulse mL/beat	11.7	6.5	(56)
Ventilatory response			
Ventilation L/min	23.8*	25.0	105
Breathing reserve		−5%	
Respiratory exchange ratio		0.80	
(*predicted from $35 \times FEV_1$)			

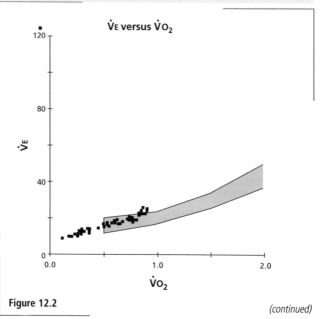

Figure 12.2

(continued)

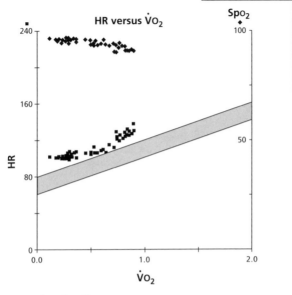

Figure 12.2 (continued)

Interpretation: His peak oxygen uptake was only 13.7 mL/kg/min, which is low (65% of predicted), even for a 71-year-old man. He stopped the test because he felt 'uncomfortable'. He did not admit to dyspnoea but grudgingly admitted some 'awareness of breathing'. His resting heart rate was high and remained higher than expected during exercise. However, he was noted to have a fine tremor, and both this and the tachycardia are probably explained by the fact that he had used multiple doses of his beta-agonist and anticholinergic inhalers before the test. Thus his heart-rate response may reflect his medication rather than cardiac disease. Against significant cardiac disease is his oxygen pulse which is appropriate for this level of exercise. His ventilatory response is initially normal but he achieves the MVV predicted by $35 \times FEV_1$ by the end of the test. His oxygen saturation falls towards the end of the test and he has no breathing reserve.

In this patient the important questions are:

- Did he try to exercise adequately? If this poor exercise tolerance is simply due to poor effort, he may still be fit enough for surgery because the measured oxygen uptake is an

underestimate. However, the cardiorespiratory responses
suggest that this was likely to be a maximal test.

- Does he have significant cardiac disease, limiting exercise? If
the exercise tolerance is limited by cardiac dysfunction, he may
still have sufficient respiratory reserves to withstand
pulmonary resection. His heart rate response is high, but this
may be due to medication. The normal oxygen-pulse response
suggests that he does not have severe cardiac dysfunction.

- Do the exercise tests demonstrate sufficient respiratory reserve
to make surgical resection of at least the right upper lobe and
possibly the entire right lung an option? In fact, the resting
lung function tests suggest advanced obstructive airways
disease, despite the fact that the DL$_{CO}$ is preserved. The
exercise response indicates that he is a high-risk candidate for
surgical resection.

The patient was advised against surgical resection and chose to
have radiotherapy treatment for his lung cancer instead.

Chapter 13

Assessing fitness to fly in patients with chronic lung disease

Air travel involves spending time in a low atmospheric pressure environment. Such an environment may be poorly tolerated by patients with chronic respiratory disease. The lung function laboratory is sometimes used to predict whether a patient is likely to develop problems during flight and whether supplemental oxygen should be used. Other aspects of medical fitness to fly are not considered here.

The flight environment

Commercial airlines are required to pressurise passenger cabins to the equivalent of a maximum altitude of about 2450 metres (8000 feet). At this level, the cabin pressure will be about 74 kPa (560 mmHg), which is 25% lower than at sea level. Although the oxygen content of the cabin air will remain at 21%, the reduction in air pressure means that the partial pressure of inspired oxygen will also fall, from 20.7 kPa (155 mmHg) at sea level to about 15 kPa (112 mmHg). This is equivalent to breathing 15% oxygen at sea level. Thus the cabin environment is not only hypobaric (low pressure), but also effectively hypoxic.

The changes in cabin pressure as an aeroplane ascends may have physiological consequences on the respiratory system. Air expands as the pressure falls. Thus a pneumothorax will worsen during flight due to expansion of the air trapped in the pleural space, and airlines refuse to carry passengers with a current or recent pneumothorax. Many people experience ear discomfort as the cabin pressure increases during the descent and the air in the middle ear is compressed. This is overcome by forcing air through the Eustachian tubes with a Valsalva manoeuvre. However, it is the effect of hypoxia that is the basis for pre-flight assessment in the lung function laboratory.

The effect of altitude on oxygenation can be predicted from the equation for the A-a gradient (see page 81). In a healthy individual with no lung disease, the partial pressure of arterial oxygen (PaO_2) when breathing 15% oxygen at sea level or normal air at an altitude of 2450 metres will fall to 7.0–8.5 kPa depending on age and minute ventilation. Because of the shape of the haemoglobin desaturation curve (see page 80), this will result in mild hypoxaemia with an arterial oxygen saturation (SaO_2) between 85% and 92%. At this level of hypoxaemia, tissue oxygen delivery will not be significantly altered and few people experience any symptoms.

The situation may be different in patients with chronic lung disease. At sea level they may already have lower partial pressure of arterial oxygen (PaO_2) due to their lung disease but, providing this remains above 8.0 kPa, they will still have relatively normal oxygen saturation (SaO_2). In an aeroplane with the cabin pressurised to 2450 metres, the fall in inspired oxygen pressure will lead to a further fall in PaO_2 and this can result in significant hypoxaemia during the flight. This may lead to dyspnoea, increasing pulmonary hypertension and increases in both the work of breathing and cardiac workload. This is potentially dangerous and flying may be hazardous for such patients. However, the number of patients who actually develop problems during flight is unknown.

Flying may be made safer by breathing supplemental oxygen during the flight, which most airlines can provide (at a cost to the patient). The issue is how to determine which patients require oxygen, how much oxygen is needed and whether some individuals are likely to become hypoxic even with supplemental oxygen so that they should avoid flying altogether.

Predicting hypoxia during flight

It is recommended that patients with chronic respiratory disease, as well as those with other conditions such as cardiac failure that may be worsened by hypoxia, undergo a pre-flight medical assessment. However, clinical assessment and simple lung function tests such as spirometry are not a reliable guide to the degree of hypoxaemia likely to be experienced in flight. Increasingly, lung function laboratories are being used to assist in this decision.

The simplest approach is to use one of several prediction equations based on the patient's PaO_2 at sea level). These have mostly been developed in COPD patients and have been shown to be reasonably reliable in this group. Based on these we can predict that patients with an arterial oxygen saturation (SaO_2) >95% do not need in-flight oxygen and that those with an SaO_2 <92% will need supplemental oxygen. Between 92% and 95%, further assessment of the severity of the underlying lung disease and the presence of other conditions is recommended. A hypoxic challenge test may be helpful to identify those who are likely to need oxygen during the flight. Patients already using oxygen at sea level are advised to increase the flow rate during flight.

Hypoxic challenge tests use a variety of methods to simulate the hypoxic environment of an aircraft cabin. These include filling a body box with a hypoxic mixture (15% O_2 = 15 kPa), using a non-rebreathing circuit and face mask delivering 15% O_2, and using either a 40% Venturi mask or a 35% Venturi mask driven by 100% nitrogen to dilute the atmospheric oxygen pressure in the entrained air to 14–15 kPa or 15–16 kPa, respectively. Commonly, the mixture is administered for 20 minutes while monitoring O_2 saturation with pulse oximetry. Most laboratories take a blood gas measurement if the SaO_2 falls below 93%.

If the PaO_2 falls below 6.6 kPa during the hypoxic challenge, it is recommended that the patient use supplemental oxygen throughout the flight or avoid flying altogether. In the range 6.6–7.5 kPa, the result is 'borderline' and some airlines' medical departments request passengers to undergo a 50-metre walk test. To 'pass' the 50-metre walk test, the patient needs to complete a 50-metre walk without distress. This is obviously a very crude measure of exercise tolerance. Pulse oximetry can be added to the test to detect major desaturation. The widely used six-minute walk or shuttle tests (see page 93) may be preferred.

It is worth pointing out that the current approach is based on common sense and knowledge of physiological principles rather than evidence. There is very little data to justify the 20-minute length of the hypoxic challenge test, the arbitrary cut-off PaO_2 of 6.6 kPa or the use of the 50-metre walk test. Airlines may be able to provide oxygen at 2 or 4 L/min only—2 L/min is probably suitable for most patients, but those already using oxygen at sea level may need a higher flow rate.

The British Thoracic Society's recommendations can be found in 'Managing passengers with respiratory disease planning air travel: British Thoracic Society recommendations', *Thorax*, 2002, 57, pp. 289–304.

CHAPTER SUMMARY

→ Aircraft are pressurised to the equivalent of no higher than 2450 metres altitude.
   – At this level, the oxygen pressure is equivalent to breathing air with only 15% (15 kPa) oxygen at sea level.
→ Assessing whether a patient with respiratory disease will tolerate this degree of hypoxia can be based on pulse oximetry at sea level.
   – Sao_2 >95%—no oxygen needed.
   – Sao_2 92–95%—supplemental oxygen may be needed depending on co-morbidity and/or response to hypoxic challenge.
   – Sao_2 <92%—in-flight oxygen recommended.
   – Using supplemental oxygen at sea level—increase oxygen flow during flight.
→ Hypoxic challenge by breathing air with 15% oxygen in the respiratory laboratory can help predict who will need in-flight oxygen.

Reference values
for spirometry

These are the 'normal' or predicted spirometric values used in most (but not all) of the examples in this book. Both prediction equations were published in 1971. The adult values (Morris, Koski & Johnson 1971) were obtained from 988 adults in Oregon, USA. Most were members of either the Church of Jesus Christ of Latter Day Saints or the Seventh Day Adventist Church, both of which forbid smoking. The children's values (Polgar & Promadhat 1971) are summary equations derived from data in several studies published by that time, and clearly oversimplify the changes in lung function occurring during growth and development.

Although both sets of prediction equations are now over 30 years old, they continue to be widely used. More recent reference values are available, but these are not necessarily any better in clinical practice. However, if local reference values are available, we suggest you use those instead.

Table A1
Predicted FEV$_1$ and FVC for adult females based on height and age (based on J. F. Morris, A. Koski & L. C. Johnson, 'Spirometric standards for healthy nonsmoking adults', *American Review of Respiratory Disease*, 103, 1971, pp. 57–67)

Age		Height (cm)								
		145	150	155	160	165	170	175	180	185
20	FEV$_1$	2.65	2.82	3.00	3.17	3.35	3.52	3.70	3.88	4.05
	FVC	3.23	3.46	3.69	3.91	4.14	4.36	4.59	4.82	5.04
25	FEV$_1$	2.52	2.70	2.87	3.05	3.22	3.40	3.57	3.75	3.93
	FVC	3.11	3.34	3.57	3.79	4.02	4.24	4.47	4.70	4.92
30	FEV$_1$	2.40	2.57	2.75	2.92	3.10	3.27	3.45	3.63	3.80
	FVC	2.99	3.22	3.45	3.67	3.90	4.12	4.35	4.58	4.80
40	FEV$_1$	2.15	2.32	2.50	2.67	2.85	3.02	3.20	3.38	3.55
	FVC	2.75	2.98	3.21	3.43	3.66	3.88	4.11	4.34	4.56
50	FEV$_1$	1.90	2.07	2.25	2.42	2.60	2.77	2.95	3.13	3.30
	FVC	2.51	2.74	2.97	3.19	3.42	3.64	3.87	4.10	4.32
60	FEV$_1$	1.65	1.82	2.00	2.17	2.35	2.52	2.70	2.88	3.05
	FVC	2.27	2.50	2.73	2.95	3.18	3.40	3.63	3.86	4.08
70	FEV$_1$	1.40	1.57	1.75	1.92	2.10	2.27	2.45	2.63	2.80
	FVC	2.03	2.26	2.49	2.71	2.94	3.16	3.39	3.62	3.84
80	FEV$_1$	1.15	1.32	1.50	1.67	1.85	2.02	2.20	2.38	2.55
	FVC	1.79	2.02	2.25	2.47	2.70	2.92	3.15	3.38	3.60

Table A2

Predicted FEV$_1$ and FVC values for adult males (based on J. F. Morris, A. Koski & L. C. Johnson, 'Spirometric standards for healthy nonsmoking adults', *American Review of Respiratory Disease*, 103, 1971, pp. 57–67)

Age		Height (cm)										
		150	155	160	165	170	175	180	185	190	195	200
20	FEV$_1$	3.53	3.71	3.90	4.08	4.26	4.44	4.62	4.80	4.98	5.16	5.34
	FVC	4.00	4.29	4.58	4.87	5.16	5.46	5.75	6.04	6.33	6.62	6.91
25	FEV$_1$	3.37	3.55	3.74	3.92	4.10	4.28	4.46	4.64	4.82	5.00	5.18
	FVC	3.87	4.17	4.46	4.75	5.04	5.33	5.62	5.91	6.20	6.50	6.79
30	FEV$_1$	3.21	3.39	3.58	3.76	3.94	4.12	4.30	4.48	4.66	4.84	5.02
	FVC	3.75	4.04	4.33	4.62	4.91	5.21	5.50	5.79	6.08	6.37	6.66
40	FEV$_1$	2.89	3.07	3.26	3.44	3.62	3.80	3.98	4.16	4.34	4.52	4.70
	FVC	3.50	3.79	4.08	4.37	4.66	4.96	5.25	5.54	5.83	6.12	6.41
50	FEV$_1$	2.57	2.75	2.94	3.12	3.30	3.48	3.66	3.84	4.02	4.20	4.38
	FVC	3.25	3.54	3.83	4.12	4.41	4.71	5.00	5.29	5.58	5.87	6.16
60	FEV$_1$	2.25	2.43	2.62	2.80	2.98	3.16	3.34	3.52	3.70	3.88	4.06
	FVC	3.00	3.29	3.58	3.87	4.16	4.46	4.75	5.04	5.33	5.62	5.91
70	FEV$_1$	1.93	2.11	2.30	2.48	2.66	2.84	3.02	3.20	3.38	3.56	3.74
	FVC	2.75	3.04	3.33	3.62	3.91	4.21	4.50	4.79	5.08	5.37	5.66
80	FEV$_1$	1.61	1.79	1.98	2.16	2.34	2.52	2.70	2.88	3.06	3.24	3.42
	FVC	2.50	2.79	3.08	3.37	3.66	3.96	4.25	4.54	4.83	5.12	5.41

Table A3

Predicted FEV$_1$ and FVC values for children based on height (based on G. Polgar & V. Promadhat, *Pulmonary Function Testing in Children: Techniques and Standards*, 1971, Philadelphia: W. B. Saunders)

Females

							Height (cm)						
	110	115	120	125	130	135	140	145	150	155	160	165	170
FEV$_1$	1.09	1.24	1.39	1.56	1.74	1.94	2.14	2.37	2.60	2.85	3.12	3.40	3.69
FVC	1.18	1.33	1.49	1.67	1.86	2.01	2.27	2.50	2.74	2.99	3.26	3.55	3.85

Males

							Height (cm)						
	110	115	120	125	130	135	140	145	150	155	160	165	170
FEV$_1$	1.09	1.24	1.39	1.56	1.74	1.94	2.14	2.37	2.60	2.85	3.12	3.40	3.69
FVC	1.25	1.41	1.58	1.75	1.94	2.15	2.36	2.60	2.84	3.10	3.38	3.67	3.97

Bibliography

Books on physiology

J. M. B. Hughes & N. B. Pride, *Lung Function Testing: Physiological Principles and Clinical Applications*, 1999, W. B. Saunders, London.

A good place to start if you want to learn more about lung function tests and physiology.

A. B. Lumb, *Nunn's Applied Respiratory Physiology*, 5th edn, 1999, Butterworth-Heinemann, Oxford.

J. B. West, *Pulmonary Pathophysiology: The Essentials*, 6th edn, 2003, Lippincott, Williams & Wilkins, Baltimore.

J. B. West, *Respiratory Physiology: The Essentials*, 7th edn, 2004, Lippincott, Williams & Wilkins, Baltimore.

Both books by West are classic student texts. Outstanding explanations of the physiology of lung function and the consequences of disease. Less useful for interpreting clinical lung function reports. The book by Lumb is an update on another classic by Nunn. This also has a long pedigree and has been particularly popular with anaesthetists.

Lung function testing

M. R. Miller, R. Crapo, J. Hankinson et al., 'General considerations for lung function testing', *European Respiratory Journal*, 2005, 26, pp. 153–61.

M. R. Miller, J. Hankinson, V. Brusasco et al., 'Standardisation of spirometry', *European Respiratory Journal*, 2005, 26, pp. 319–38.

R. Pellegrino, G. Viegi, P. Enright et al., 'Interpretative strategies for lung function tests', *European Respiratory Journal*, 2005, 26(5).

These articles, and others in the series published in the European Respiratory Journal, are the result of an American Thoracic Society and European Respiratory Society joint task force on standardisation of lung function testing.

D. Johns & R. Pierce, *McGraw-Hill's Pocket Guide to Spirometry*, 2003, McGraw-Hill, Sydney.

G. L. Ruppel, *Manual of Pulmonary Function Testing*, 8th edn, 2003, Mosby-Year Book, Inc., St Louis.

An outstanding manual of how to perform lung function tests. Comprehensive.

http://www.spirxpert.com

A useful website on spirometry by P. H. Quanjer.

Exercise testing

European Respiratory Society, 'Clinical exercise testing with reference to lung diseases: indications, standardization and interpretation strategies', *European Respiratory Journal*, 1997, 10, pp. 2662–89.

'ATS/ACCP statement on cardiopulmonary exercise testing', *American Journal of Respiratory and Critical Care Medicine*, 2003, 167, pp. 211–77.

'ATS statement: guidelines for the six-minute walk test', *American Journal of Respiratory and Critical Care Medicine*, 2002, 166, pp. 111–17.

K. Wasserman, J. E. Hansen, D. Y. Sue, W. W. Stringer & B. J. Whipp, *Principles of Exercise Testing & Interpretation: Including Pathophysiology and Clinical Applications*, 4th edn, 2004, Lippincott, Williams & Wilkins, Baltimore.

N. L. Jones, *Clinical Exercise Testing*, 4th edn, 1997, W. B. Saunders, Philadelphia.

Both excellent books which offer different perspectives on exercise tests.

Other lung function tests

'ATS/ERS recommendations for standardized procedures for the online and offline measurement of exhaled lower respiratory nitric oxide and nasal nitric oxide, 2005', *American Journal of Respiratory and Critical Care Medicine*, 2005, 171, pp. 912–30.

'ATS/ERS statement on respiratory muscle testing', *American Journal of Respiratory and Critical Care Medicine*, 2002, 166, pp. 518–624.

ERS Task Force, 'The forced oscillation technique in clinical practice: methodology, recommendations and future developments', *European Respiratory Journal*, 2003, 22, pp. 1026–41.

Assessing patients for thoracic resection

British Thoracic Society and Society of Cardiothoracic Surgeons of Great Britain and Ireland, 'Guidelines on the selection of patients with lung cancer for surgery', *Thorax*, 2001, 56, pp. 89–108. Also available on the British Thoracic Society website, www.brit-thoracic.org.uk.

Assessing fitness to fly

'Managing passengers with respiratory disease planning air travel: British Thoracic Society recommendations', *Thorax*, 2002, 57, pp. 289–304.

Other resources

National and international respiratory societies often produce updates and standardisation statements on lung function testing. See the websites listed below. It is also worth looking up other societies, particularly your local society.

Websites

American Thoracic Society: www.thoracic.org
British Thoracic Society: www.brit-thoracic.org.uk
European Respiratory Society: www.ersnet.org
Thoracic Society of Australia & New Zealand: www.thoracic.org.au

Index

Page numbers in **bold** print refer to main entries, while page numbers in *italic* refer to figures and tables. Clinical examples are indexed by chapter topic only. All abbreviations used in the index can be found on pages x–xiv.